WHEELING AROUND LOUISVILLE

D1500850

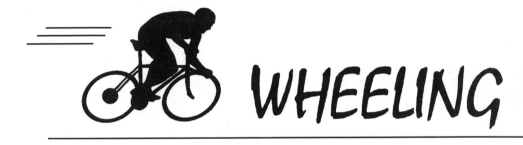

WHEELING

Joe Ward's

AROUND LOUISVILLE

25 Great Bike Rides
Around Louisville, Jefferson County
and Southern Indiana

Happy trails –

Joe Ward

Butler Books
Louisville

To Gil Morris, who preserved the traditions through the lean years.

Published by Butler Books
P.O. Box 7311
Louisville, KY 40207

ISBN 1-884532-44-6

Printed in Canada

TABLE OF CONTENTS

INTRODUCTION

I wrote this book to encourage you to ride your bicycle. It will be good for you, and for the world. You will get a little exercise on even the shortest rides, and a lot of good exercise on the longer ones. You will get a different view of an interesting region, and it will improve your understanding and outlook. And while you're riding, you won't be driving your car.

What I'd like you to do with this book is read through the narratives while looking at the maps and route sheets. Photocopy the maps and route sheets if necessary, so you can put them side by side and make it easier. You'll want the copies anyway, to put on your stem clip while you ride. If you don't have a stem clip, I'll tell you how to make one toward the end of this section. (See page 9.)

Look a route over well, getting a good idea where the turns are, and of sites along the way that you might want to pay special attention to. Then go ride it.

Some people prefer route sheets, which just say where to turn. But I've always liked maps. They give you an idea at a glance where you are in relation to other parts of the ride. When I started riding almost 30 years ago, cyclists liked handlebar bags, and there usually was a map case on top of the bag, where you'd put a map for handy reference as you rode along. Such bags aren't used as much these days, but the clip works just as well.

My idea for this book was to make both maps and route sheets the right size, so that a direct photo copy, with a little trimming would be right for the clip – not so big they'd be too floppy, and not so small that you couldn't read them. If you clip in both a map and a route sheet, though, don't get to fiddling with them and run off the road or come to other calamity.

I arranged the rides in the book for the most part with beginning riders in mind, people who mostly ride around the neighborhood. I start with short, easy rides, and work up to some fairly substantial ones at the end. If you're a beginner, you should take them in that order, improving your strength and abilities as you go. But even experienced riders should find rides they'll like at both ends of the book.

The first few are what the Louisville Bicycle Club used to call "Turtle Rides" – so named to counter a notion beginning riders sometimes get that club members will ride off and leave them in the dust.

Turtlemistress Marilyn Minnick decreed that Turtle Rides be 10 miles long or thereabouts, have no hills, and be undertaken at a slow pace. Marilyn says she got the idea from another club's newsletter.

You can take these Turtle Rides at any pace you like, but they otherwise generally meet the criteria. If they seem a bit convoluted in some cases, it's because it's not always easy to put together 10 continuous miles in Louisville without encountering hills. Downtown, where it is essentially flat otherwise, there are a lot of underpasses. I've also tried to shun busier streets, and to route you by buildings and other objects that are interesting to know about.

It should be noted that downtown rides, especially, are most enjoyable when undertaken fairly early on a weekend morning. There's not much traffic downtown then, and you can pretty much cycle along and gawk at your leisure. The downtown rides probably are not much fun at all during morning or afternoon rush hour. But I have ridden downtown a lot in the middle of the afternoon and enjoyed it quite a bit.

The Turtle Rides are starter rides, intended to give you an idea how much fun it is to get out of your car and pedal out onto the streets. If you have much experience as a cyclist at all, you'll find them short. If you're just beginning to ride, you may not know it yet, but you, too, soon will find them too short, and you'll be wanting longer rides.

There are some pretty long rides later in the book. But you should note that the shorter rides can be strung together as well, or combined with alternatives you devise yourself. For in-town riding, a good city map – such as the one published by AAA Kentucky – is a good place to look for streets that can be added on.

And that is fitting, because the American Automobile Club, of which AAA Kentucky in Louisville is an affiliate, is a surviving arm of a bicycle touring and racing organization begun in 1880 and called the League of American Wheelmen.

I got interested in cycling because of its environmental and health connections in the late 1960s, when I was the environmental writer for *The Courier-Journal*. Like a lot of people interested for those reasons, I kind of gave it lip service for several years. I did buy a couple of bicycles and ride them, but I didn't know what I was doing, and I didn't ride much.

Then one day in the early 1970s, when I was working in the newspaper's Bluegrass Bureau in Lexington, I decided to go on a ride with the Bluegrass

Wheelmen, as the Lexington bike club was then called, and write about it.

I showed up looking ridiculous on a bike much too small for me. I was wearing blue jeans, which are tight and stiff and make riding harder because they bind at the hips, and tennis shoes, which lack the stiff sole needed to keep the pedals from making your feet numb.

Who knew? Bikes were advertised by department stores, then as now, as though one size fits all. I'm 6' 5" and I was riding a bike designed for somebody a foot or more shorter. It does make a difference. You can't get your stride on a bike that's too small. It's like trying to hike in a duck-walking crouch. And on a bike that's too big, of course, you can hurt yourself.

I couldn't begin to keep up with the Lexington group on even a short ride, and I didn't think bicycling was very much fun. But, a couple of the members told me as gently as they could what I was doing wrong.

I saved my money, and in the summer of 1975 bought a beautiful blue Schwinn LeTour bicycle, which was lightweight and had a frame that was big enough for me. I thought I'd died and gone to heaven. I started riding to work, and found I couldn't go straight home. I'd sometimes take a couple of hours cycling around Lexington after work.

Before too long, my bureau partner Doug Perry and I rode our bikes from Lexington to Louisville and wrote about it for the paper. I was seriously hooked. I moved back to the C-J's features department in Louisville in 1977, and began riding my bike to work on days when I didn't need my car for a story.

I kept careful track of my commuting miles. On July 3, 1990, as I cycled past what is now Distillery Commons on Lexington Road, I passed 24,901.55 miles, equivalent to the circumference of the earth at the equator. I've been around at least once more since.

While I was doing that, I got interested in Effective Cycling, a concept then promoted by Californian John Forester and the League of American Wheelmen – another surviving arm of that 1880 cycling league. I became a cycling instructor certified by the league, which is now called the League of American Bicyclists.

Some Suggestions

* For the kind of riding I suggest in this book, a road bike is best. That is, a

bike with narrow 27-inch or 700c wheels, and drop handlebars. Mountain bikes would do for some of the short rides, but they'd be less fun for anything over 15 or 16 miles. Their fat tires have a lot of rolling resistance, and their straight handlebars encourage an upright riding posture that makes for a sore posterior before long.

The secret of riding the skinny saddles found on road bikes, incidentally, is weight distribution. Only about one third of your weight should be on the saddle, with another third on the pedals and the remaining third on the handlebars. Bear down on your pedals and raise up off your saddle slightly once in awhile until weight distribution becomes automatic.

Padded cycling shorts help, as do cycling gloves with padded leather palms that absorb handlebar shock and protect your hands in the case of a fall.

* You should wear a helmet if you ride bicycles. Unless you're on a recumbent, the distance from your skull to the pavement when you're astride a bicycle is enough to crack your head in a straight fall. Helmets are available in a bewildering assortment. Make sure it's CPSC certified, but you don't have to pay a lot of money. The important thing is your head.

* You will likely need some sort of bike rack for your car to do many of these rides, unless you have a vehicle large enough to haul a bike or two. You also will need a tire patch kit, a set of tire irons, and a frame-mounted tire pump. The thin tires on road bicycles unfortunately do puncture easily, and if you don't have the right equipment and skill to patch a tire, your range will be fairly limited.

 * About that stem clip. It goes on the stem of your bicycle – that arm that comes out of the frame and holds onto your handlebars. It's easy to make yourself. Get a small binder-type paper clip – the kind made of flat, black metal with wire bails. Fasten one of the bails to the stem of your bicycle so that the clip opens toward the saddle.

Use a nylon tie fastener, the kind with a sort of ratchet edge that will hold the clip snugly once you pull it tight. Trim off the loose end and wrap a neat piece of plastic tape around tie fastener and wire bail. You use the free bail to pry the clip open and let it snap shut.

* I found early on in my cycling that an odometer adds to the enjoyment. It's fun to know how far you've gone. A word of warning, though. One of the first things we noticed when electronic odometers became readily available is that five riders could start out at the same time, all set at zero, and after a mile and a half, none of their odometers would agree.

I give mileage to the tenth of a mile on route sheets for this book, but don't expect yours to match exactly. The mileage figures are more of a ballpark sort of thing, intended to alert you if you should get a mile or two off the course.

Bike equipment is available from bike shops, online or from catalogs. Some good Louisville-area bicycle shops, presented here in alphabetical order, include:
Bardstown Road Bicycles, 1051 Bardstown Rd., 485-9795
Bicycle Sport, 128 Breckenridge Lane, 897-2611
Clarksville Schwinn & Fitness, 111 W. Hwy. 31, Clarksville, 948-2453
Derby City Outfitters, 960 Baxter Ave., 589-9055
Dixie Schwinn Cyclery, 1803 Rockford Lane, 448-3448
Highland Cycle, 1737 Bardstown Rd., 458-7832
Jeffersonville Schwinn & Fitness, 1537 E. 10th St., Jeffersonville, 284-2453
St. Matthews Schwinn Cyclery & Fitness, 106 Sears Ave., 895-0553
Scheller's Fitness & Cycling, 11520 Shelbyville Rd., 245-1955, and 8323 Preston Hwy., 969-4100

* It's often fun to ride by yourself or with a small group of your own choosing, but there's a good bit of enjoyment to be had riding with a bicycle club, too. You can learn a lot about riding almost by osmosis while riding with a club, and if you want to build your conditioning so you can do longer trips, you can usually find the kind of challenge you need with club riders.

The Louisville-area has two big bike clubs that do rides like those in this book – in fact, they ride on all of the actual roads in this book. They are the Louisville Bicycle Club, formerly the Louisville Wheelmen, and the Southern Indiana Wheelmen, or SIW. The Slow Spokes is a subgroup of the Southern Indiana club, formed to invite people looking for a more leisurely pace.

The Louisville group also has rides aimed at more sedate riders, and they were called Rif Raf rides at this writing, sort of an evolution from Turtle Rides. The Louisville Club has another group on the other end of that spectrum – people who like to do 100 miles rides in January and such. They call themselves the Mad Dogs.

Both main clubs list their ride schedules online – at http://www.louisvillebicycleclub.org/touring.htm for the Louisville club and http://members.aye.net/~siw/ride_schedules/index.html for the Southern Indiana group. Ride schedules also are available in bike shops.

As you ride roads in the area, you are likely to see their ride markings at intersections – sometimes in such profusion that it's impossible to tell which ride goes where. The most common marking is a Dan Henry arrow, named for its presumed inventor, a long-time member of the League of American Bicyclists.

It's a circle with a pointer, usually put on the pavement in white spray paint. A good one looks like this:

*Dogs can be a problem for cyclists, especially out in the country. A lot of riders think there is more danger that they'll run out in front of a bicycle, causing a wreck, than that they'll bite. I've seen a very small dog bring a very strong rider down, and it wasn't pretty. And I've been bitten myself, and didn't care for that, either.

Cyclists have tried all sorts of defenses. I often try talking softly – "Hi, dog. Nice dog." And if that doesn't work, speak sternly. "No! Lie down!" Once I found a group of dogs way out in the country that would not respond to "Lie down!" but seemed to understand "Lay down!" quite well. I know some teachers who find they can be effective if they yell really loudly.

It's dangerous to swing at a dog with a tire pump, because it can throw you off balance, or the pump can end up in your spokes. Some riders squirt dogs with water bottles, with good effect. But you'd have to be in good control of your bike to do that without danger.

One thing I've found that seems to work fairly consistently is a bell. You can buy a handlebar or stem-mounted bell at a bike shop. When I see a dog that's likely to chase – if he's chased riders ahead of me, for example – I start ringing the bell rapidly and repeatedly as I come into his territory. The ringing seems to confuse dogs momentarily, and usually a slight hesitation by the dog gives you a chance to be gone.

If you are bitten, and it's safe to do so, you should stop and talk to the dog's owner. Find out if the dog has had its shots. And, in any case, you should contact health authorities in the county where the dog lives. They may want to quarantine him, or take other action.

* Finally, you should be at least a little bit aware of the aforementioned Effective Cycling, which is a sort of cycling discipline, also known as vehicular cycling, based on lore from generations of riders in England. It's the basis for a League of American Bicyclists education program now called Bike Ed.

A book called Effective Cycling is the "bible" of the discipline, written by John Forester, a California cycling authority, and published by MIT Press. It includes a lot of information on how bicycles work, how to maintain them, and how to ride them safely. It usually costs about $32.50, and I recommend it highly for anybody who wants to know about cycling.

The mantra of vehicular cycling is, "Bicyclists fare best when they act and are treated as drivers of vehicles." All the states now view bicycles as vehicles, and afford them the same general rights as other vehicles, while requiring them to meet the same general responsibilities.

For a thorough understanding of Effective Cycling you need Forester's book. But basically, it amounts to riding your bike – or driving it, as Forester likes to say – the same way you would drive your car.

You ride in the same direction as motor traffic, not facing it as a pedestrian would. And you don't ride on the sidewalk. That's a visibility matter. The driver of a car pulling up to an intersection looks out in to the traffic lanes for conflicting traffic before going ahead.

He doesn't expect anything faster than pedestrian traffic on the sidewalk, so if you are zipping along there, he is likely to either hit you or pull out in front of you. He won't see you riding along close to the curb in the opposite direction of motor traffic, either.

You obey traffic signals just as you would in a car, and yield to cross traffic where it has the right of way. When you are riding on a minor street that intersects a major one, you look for traffic from both directions, and proceed when the way is clear.

You position yourself on lanes according to your intention at an intersection. When you're driving your car, if you intend to turn left at an intersection, you move into the left lane first. It's essentially the same for a bicycle.

Vehicular cyclists actually treat each lane as if it were two. When preparing for a left turn, for example, you move from the right side of the right lane to the left side of it. Then move from the left side of that lane to the right side of the next lane, and so forth, in careful steps.

As you would in a car, you yield to traffic behind you when changing lanes, checking carefully to be sure the lane is clear before moving into it. And use hand signals, the same ones people used to use in cars, except that a right turn can be signaled with the right arm held straight out.

A right turn is made from the right side of the right lane. If you plan to go straight through an intersection, you would move to the left side of the right lane, so drivers behind you know you will not turn.

Most traffic lanes have plenty of room for a car and a bike to travel safely side by side. Some don't, though — there may be parked cars, or some other obstruction.

If a lane is too narrow for side-by-side safety, you wait until the lane is clear of traffic close behind you, and then move out far enough in the lane so that drivers behind you will stay behind you — rather than trying to squeeze past — until it is safe for them to pass.

Ride far enough out into the street so that if the door of a parked car were suddenly thrown open, you wouldn't smash into it. That happens to inexperienced riders all the time. Also watch for debris and other hazards — such as drain grates — close along the curb. Don't ride in the line of broken glass and small rocks that spinning automobile tires sweep to the curb.

A lot of effective cycling is just thinking ahead — watching traffic both ahead of you and behind you, and moving to the place you need to be before you're in conflict with another driver.

You can communicate with drivers, and negotiate with them, by looking at them and looking at a spot you'd like to move into. I've seen many courtesies from car drivers in my years of commuting through downtown Louisville. They just want to know what to expect from you.

Position yourself in the lane according to speed, as you would in your car — faster traffic to the left, slower traffic to the right. Pass slower traffic on the left.

Well, that's the gist of it. Travel by bicycle is travel in human scale. You're at ground level. You feel the breeze and smell the flowers. You hear the birds. Sometimes as I'd ride in to work in the morning along Muhammad Ali Boulevard, I'd pass some small girls swinging their jump rope, singing their jump rope songs. I was really glad I wasn't in a car.

It's the same out in the countryside. On a bike, it's easy to stop anywhere. Finding a place to pull off is not a problem. You can take that picture. If your daughter's with you, she can pet that horse. You can sometimes make out the inscription on that old tombstone. And if there's a person out in the field or on the lawn, you can stop and ask questions.

Or you can just whiz along, over hill and dale, listening to the whisper of your wheels on the pavement.

Enjoy these rides.

WHEELING AROUND LOUISVILLE

25 Great Bike Rides
Around Louisville, Jefferson County
and Southern Indiana

Tour de Nabes

10 miles

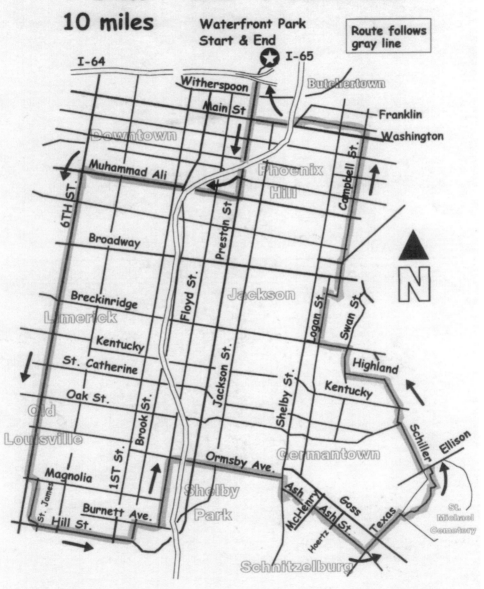

Waterfront Park
Start & End

Route follows
gray line

I-64

I-65

Witherspoon

Butchertown

Main St

Franklin

Downtown

Washington

Muhammad Ali

Phoenix Hill

6TH ST.

Campbell St.

N

Broadway

Preston St.

Jackson

Breckinridge

Floyd St.

Logan St.

Swan St.

Limerick

Kentucky

Highland

St. Catherine

Jackson St.

Kentucky

Oak St.

Shelby St.

Old
Louisville

1ST St.

Brook St.

Ormsby Ave.

Germantown

Schiller

Ellison

Magnolia

St. James

Shelby
Park

Ash

McHenry

Goss

Texas

St. Michael
Cemetery

Burnett Ave.

Ash St.

Hill St.

Hoertz

Schnitzelburg

Tour de Nabes

Turtle Ride. Ten miles. No hills. Potential traffic on some streets. Start at Waterfront Park, off River Road near Preston Street.

Louisville is a great place for neighborhoods, and this ride was designed to give you a feel for a handful of them in an hour or two, depending on how much you want to gawk around. I like to take this one easy, myself.

And it is a Turtle Ride, a name the club used for a time for rides intended to attract new riders, with a promise that the ride would be short and have no hills, and that the pace would be slow.

Downtown

Starting at **Waterfront Park**, you pull out onto River Road, then keep going straight on Preston Street at the first stoplight. River Road turns right, but you'll go straight, up past **Louisville Slugger Field** on your left. More about that later. You keep going, staying toward the right edge of the street, to turn right on Muhammad Ali Boulevard, and stay to the right along here.

You're cycling right through the heart of downtown Louisville now. And the neighborhood, appropriately, is called "Downtown." That building on the left after you pass Third Street is the **Pendennis Club**, seat of generations of Louisville movers and shakers. At Fourth Street you pass the **Seelbach Hotel**, a dowager restored to former elegance, on the left, and the Galleria, engine of downtown renewal, on the right.

Safety Note: You should be thinking about getting across to the left side of the street anywhere along here. Remember your vehicular cycling drill: glance back, move half a lane to the left, straighten up, check back again, etc. until you're in the left side of the left-most lane. (See page 12.)

Turn left onto Sixth Street. You'll have the light, so it's okay to cross right over to the right side of the street and proceed South. At Broadway notice the 1950-era **Courier-Journal building** on your left – Louisville's famous "Wind Tunnel at Sixth and Broadway."

Limerick

When you pass Breckinridge Street, you are in the **Limerick** neighborhood, once the home of Irish families whose breadwinners worked in the rail yards a couple of blocks west. This chunk of Sixth Street used to come alive with an annual St. Patrick's Day Parade that ran from **St. Louis**

17

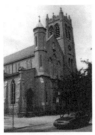
Bertrand Catholic Church up to Broadway, from the 1860s until 1918. The imposing stone church building dates to 1872. Before you get to that, though, notice the distinctive brick building on the Southeast corner of Sixth and Breckinridge. That was the old **Central Colored School**, opened in 1873, thought to be the first tax-supported public school for African Americans in the state.

St. Louis Bertrand

Old Louisville

From Limerick you pass into the **Old Louisville** neighborhood. Nothing exemplifies the Victorian splendor of Old Louisville more than **St. James Court**, so we turn left on Magnolia Street and then hang a right onto the Court. Many of those magnificent old houses are open for tours during the fall holidays.

At Hill Street we turn left again, taking the right side of the outside lane. Hill Street can be busy, depending on time of day, so be careful. We're only going a few blocks. We've reached one of the convolutions intended to keep the route flat – by avoiding the Hill Street underpass. We turn left on Brook Street, then jog right on Burnett Avenue to Floyd Street, for a little less traffic. We're still seeing the great churches and Victorian houses of Old Louisville here.

Shelby Park

At Ormsby Avenue, we turn right and duck under I-65, passing into the **Shelby Park** neighborhood. Those are authentic shotgun houses along there, mostly built before 1910. Supposedly, they are so-named because they put one room behind another, and a shotgun blast into the front door could make it out the back without hitting anything. One school of thought is that they were built long and skinny to fit narrow urban lots, for tax purposes.

Schnitzelburg

We turn right onto Shelby Street, and move left in the lane so we can turn left as soon as we pass the barrier in the center of the street. Our objective is Ash Street, but we have to go a short distance past it because of the barrier. We turn left into an alley, then left immediately into another alley, then right onto Ash Street. We are briefly in the **Schnitzelburg** neighborhood, home of the **World Championship Dainty Contest**. Dainty is a neighborhood game that involves whacking a short, pointed length of broomstick with a longer length of broomstick, so that it pops up into the air, and then trying to knock the airborne chunk as far as you can. I've never been hit by a flying dainty here.

But you can take a little side trip a block left on Hoertz Avenue to see the marks on the street by which they measure distances achieved. The route doesn't go that way, though, because that would put you on Goss Avenue, a fairly busy street.

Before Hoertz, though, we take a jog at McHenry Street, and stay on Ash. Some riders may note a slight acclivity on Ash Street at this point. (ac·cliv·i·ty: *n.* An upward slope, as of a hill). But this is not a hill. There are no hills on these Turtle Rides, remember? No hills.

No uphills, anyway. Turn left on Texas Street and head down toward **St. Michael Cemetery**. Downhills are permitted on Turtle Rides, and here's one. You may even say, "yippee," if you like. You're on Texas, after all.

Germantown

But be respectful once you enter **St. Michael Cemetery**. A cemetery is a great place to learn things, by reading tombstones, and there is no better way to tour a cemetery than by bicycle, especially if it is a large cemetery.

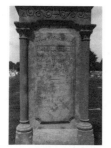
Some cemeteries exclude cyclists, though, presumably on the mistaken impression that a cyclist is likely to be a vandal, and we don't want to add to that perception. If you look closely at some of the stones in St. Michael's, you'll learn that you're now in the Germantown neighborhood, because some inscriptions are in German.

You can wander around as long as you want to in the cemetery. It's peaceful and there's no traffic. If you wander around enough, you may find the grave of "Samson" – actor **Victor Mature**, a Louisville native who died and was buried here in 1999.

If you don't want to wander, just take every right turn you get a chance to, starting just inside the Texas Street entrance, and you'll find your way out the other gate. Keep watching on your left and you'll see Mature's white, very theatrical gravestone about a third of the way through.

Turn left onto Ellison Avenue and go a short distance to Schiller Avenue. Enjoy the slight downhill there and ignore what might be the optical illusion of an acclivitous stretch up to Oak Street. You bear left there a little through the light to continue on Schiller, and you pass the imposing twin steeples of **St. Therese Little Flower of Jesus Catholic Church** at Kentucky.

It's a Germantown landmark, though the architectural style is Spanish Baroque. Stay on Schiller to a left on Highland, then a right on Swan.

Buy Stuff
Swan Street is home to the **Come Back Inn**, where you can get very good food at reasonable prices, and beer. Be sure to lock up your bikes if you leave them outside, though. Better yet, ask if there is somewhere to stash them out of sight. The old Swan Street Antique Mall, which used to be catty-corner across Swan and Breckinridge, was a great place for bargains in furniture and doodads. It has closed, alas.

Smoketown
A left on Breckinridge takes you down to Logan Street and a right turn. You're in the **Smoketown–Jackson** neighborhood, thought to have taken its name from the chimneys of numerous brick kilns to be found in the area as early as the 1820s. Many of the brick workers were blacks, and Smoketown may be the only Louisville neighborhood where African Americans have lived continuously since before the Civil War.

Phoenix Hill
Follow Logan to Finzer Street, and jog right and then left onto Campbell Street. Across Broadway, work your way into the left lane and keep going straight where Gray Street crosses. A car can't go straight there because of a barrier, but you can. You get up on the sidewalk that is straight ahead, for a short space. It's just one of the perks of being on a bicycle. Be careful of the curb as you get off. I'd walk.

You're in the **Phoenix Hill** neighborhood now. A chunk of the neighborhood, up toward Baxter Avenue and Broadway, used to be the site of **Phoenix Hill Park** and the **Phoenix Hill Brewery**, altogether a place of great partying in the late 1800s and early 1900s. That Castle-like building on the right as you pass Liberty Street was home to the old **Moll Lumber Co.**, from the 1930s.

Butchertown
Crossing Main Street, you enter **Butchertown**, another German neighborhood that thrived as a center of meat production from the 1820s into the early part of this century. Turn left onto Washington Street, then left again on Hancock Street, and right onto Main Street.

There you see **Louisville Slugger Field**, a very nice 13,000-seat "retro classic" minor league baseball park built in an old train shed, as part of the revitalization of Louisville's riverfront area. The bronze statue out front depicts **Harold Henry "Pee Wee" Reese**, the great Dodger shortstop, who smoothed Jackie Robinson's way into the big leagues in 1947.

Safety Note: Turn right on Preston and back to the park. Remember your vehicular cycling as you move to the left side of the left lane to turn into the parking lot.

Route Sheet

Start, Waterfront Park
0.0   Right on River Road
0.2   Straight on Preston
0.8   Right on Muhammad Ali
1.6   Left on Sixth
3.2   Left on Magnolia
3.3   Right on St. James
3.5   Left on Hill
4.0   Left on Brook
4.1   Right on Burnett
4.2   Left on Floyd
4.6   Right on Ormsby
4.7   Jog right at Preston, left on Ormsby
5.1   Right on Shelby
5.2   Left around barrier into alley, then left into another alley, then right on Ash
5.3   Jog left on McHenry, right on Ash
5.7   Left on Texas
6.0   Enter St. Michael Cemetery; Bear right after the gate, then take the first left between Sections B and C, then the first right between Sections G and E, then turn left at the Section H marker. Stay straight across a road, then take two lefts and a right out the gate
6.5   Left on Ellison and right on Schiller
6.8   Left on Oak, right on Schiller, cross Kentucky and bear left on Schiller
7.0   Left on Highland
7.2   Right on Swan
7.3   Left on Breckinridge
7.4   Right on Logan
7.7   Right on Finzer, left on Campbell
7.9   Get in left lane, take a short stretch of sidewalk straight ahead, straight on Campbell
8.6   Left on Washington
9.0   Left on Hancock and right on Main
9.4   Right on Preston
9.9   Back at Park

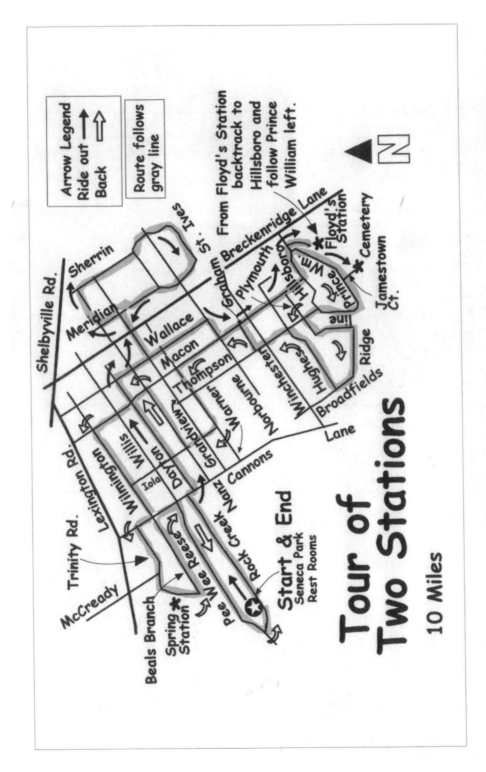

Tour of Two Stations

10 Miles

Tour of Two Stations

Turtle Ride. Ten miles. No hills. Start at the Seneca Park rest rooms, along Rock Creek Road, half a mile from Cannons Lane.

This is another Turtle Ride, designed to be short and flat and offer landmarks of interest. I was surprised to find, when I started exploring for Turtle Rides, that it's not really easy to find 10 miles of street with no hills, especially east of downtown. Sometimes it took real ingenuity to work it out.

Then when I started mapping the routes, I found that, on a map, ingenuity can look like quite the bewildering swirl. The main problem is that I had to use short stretches of Grandview and Macon Avenues twice – once on the way out and once on the way back – to catch a traffic light and to avoid hills.

I've tried to reduce the confusion by using solid arrows for the outbound trip and outlined arrows for the trip back. Still, it helps to study this map a little, and to refer to the route sheet where the map is puzzling.

It's a nice little ride, though, great for a summer evening. Beside passing two 18th Century stations, where our forebears huddled together for protection against Indians during the Revolutionary War, it goes through some neighborhoods and small cities that I believe represent suburbia at its best.

You can get a feeling on this route, on a summer afternoon, that you're about to be overcome by charcoal starter fumes. Once, on Hughes Road, I saw a pretty young woman walking FIVE golden retrievers.

Vintage Subdivisions

Start at the parking lot by the restrooms near the **Seneca Park** playing fields. Ride out Rock Creek Road and jog right, then left, across Cannons Lane onto Dayton Avenue. Notice the architecture of the houses along here. They definitely are of a period. People flocked to the high ground here after the 1937 flood, and kept coming after World War II.

Hang a right at Wallace Avenue and head south, then turn left on Grandview Avenue and cross Breckenridge Lane. Take a left on Meridian Avenue, a right on Nanz Avenue, and another right on Sherrin Ave. Then go straight awhile, right through a narrow gate just after you pass Hycliffe Avenue.

By the time you get down to **St. Germaine Court**, where you take a left and follow the circle across Norbourne Boulevard, you'll notice subtly different architecture from that along Dayton. The period appears to be about the same, but here more houses have a second story, and front doors tend to be a bit more ornate.

Sam Thomas, Louisville historian and historic preservation afficionado, told me it was mostly a difference in the vision of the architects and developers.

Follow St. Ives Court around and cross Norbourne again, and turn left on Meridian Ave.

Off Road Stuff

Meridian is more of a suggestion than an actual street in places. You will proceed through another narrow gate, then bear right at the end of Warner Avenue onto a paved path that follows a line of bushes just west of **St. Matthews City Hall**. Follow that onto Grandview, hang a left to re-cross Breckenridge, and then turn left again on Wallace. Go right at Norbourne to avoid **Our Lady of Lourdes Elementary School**, but take a left on Macon Avenue to keep heading toward **Floyd's Station**.

Old Fort

At Hillsboro Court go left, and take the driveway into the **Jamestown Apartment** complex. It's private property. The sign asks you not to solicit.

Follow the driveway back to the right. Beyond the end of the parking lot, you'll see the remains of an old stone well house.

It's what's left of a **stockade built in 1779 by Col. John Floyd**, one of six stations that dotted the middle fork of Beargrass Creek out from the Falls of the Ohio in Louisville's earliest days.

Floyd and his family and neighbors crowded into the station there from time to time in the couple of years after it was built, while Indians who had been stirred up by the British picked off people around the community. Accounts suggest the close quarters made people sick and cranky.

Col. Floyd's Grave

Backtrack out of the complex and go left again on Prince William

Street. Turn left into Jamestown Court and stop and look over the wall into the cemetery there. **John Floyd** is buried there, with some members of his family. He ultimately was killed by Indians, at age 33 in 1783, but he'd had an amazing career by then.

He'd surveyed land near the falls in 1774, had participated in the rescue of the Callaway girls and Jemima Boone near Boonesborough in 1776, had preyed on British shipping on the high seas in a privateer, and escaped from a British prison and made his way back to Virginia – all before he brought his wife and baby out to Kentucky to set up the station.

He marched with Gen. George Rogers Clark, was named commander of the Jefferson County Militia, and was a judge.

The Indians got him on his way to Bullitt's Lick one day.

One of his sons and also a grandson became governor of Virginia, and the German count whose land was confiscated during World War I for Bowman Field was one of his progeny. His nephew, Sgt. Charles Floyd, was the only member of the 1803-1806 Lewis and Clark expedition to the west coast who died during the trip. Historians believe appendicitis killed him.

Suburbia at Its Best

Take Prince William on around. It becomes Hillsboro Court at some point, and the route turns left onto Thompson Avenue, and left again a short block later onto Plymouth Road. Take a left shortly onto Ridgeline Drive, and follow it around to the right.

You will say there are hills on Ridgeline, and it is true, in a sense. They actually are whoop-de-dos, picked by me deliberately to show Turtle Riders that if you pedal briskly down an incline, you sometimes can actually coast up the other side. So they don't really count as hills.

Turn right onto Hughes Road. Note that the architecture has changed again. Turn left on Thompson again, then right on Graham Road and left on Macon. That is all to miss slight hills. We aim to pamper.

You leave Macon again at Warner Avenue, follow it to a right on Iola, a right on Nanz Avenue, and a left on Macon again. That's all to add a little distance. This is a very short ride as it is. We didn't want Turtle Riders to feel like wimps.

Safety Note: Macon crosses Willis Avenue, a through street on which traffic can get moving pretty fast in either direction. Scofflaws. Be careful crossing there, and turn left on Wilmington Avenue.

Spring Station

Turn right on Cannons Lane and make a quick left on Trinity Road. Bear right onto McCready Avenue, and then make a left back onto Trinity – where you can read a historic marker about **Spring Station**, another of the Beargrass forts.

While you're stopped at the sign, try to get a look through the trees ahead and to the left at a mansion also called Spring Station, which was restored in the late 1970s by movie star Roger Davis.

The restored stone spring house that marks the location of the old fort is on the right, a few tenths of a mile on down Trinity.

Beal's Branch

Spring Station was built by 1780 and served pioneers through the same perilous times their neighbors weathered up the creek a way. A Virginia merchant named Samuel Beall bought the station and nearby land about 1784. His son, Norborne Booth Beall, started the house that eventually became the current mansion about 1802.

Water still flows out of the spring at Spring Station—you can see it bubbling up out of the ground behind the spring house—and it forms **Beals Branch**, which flows into Beargrass Creek. Apparently spelling wasn't considered a big deal in the days when it was named.

Hang a left on the street named for the branch, and follow it back to Cannons Lane. Turn right, then right again on Pee Wee Reese Road, and follow that around the playing fields to a left on Rock Creek, back to the starting point.

Route Sheet

Start at the Seneca Park restrooms on Rock Creek Drive

0.0	Proceed on Rock Creek to Cannons Lane
0.5	Jog right on Cannons, left on Dayton
1.0	Right on Wallace
1.3	Left on Grandview
1.4	Cross Breckenridge, turn left on Meridian
1.5	Right on Nanz
1.7	Right on Sherrin
2.0	Left on Germaine Court-Sherrin, follow it across Norbourne and around to the right on St. Ives Court
2.5	Cross Norbourne again
2.6	Left on Meridian through gate
2.8	Bear right at the end of Warner, onto paved path, then turn left onto Grandview, and re-cross Breckenridge
3.0	Left on Wallace
3.4	Right on Norbourne
3.5	Left on Macon
3.9	Left on Hillsboro
4.1	Right into Jamestown apartments
4.2	Spring house. Retrace path to Hillsboro
4.4	Left on Hillsboro and left on Prince William
4.7	Left into Jamestown Court and back out, left on Prince William, and follow around to right, where it becomes Hillsboro.
5.2	Left on Thompson, left on Plymouth
5.3	Left on Ridgeline
5.7	Right on Hughes
6.0	Left on Thompson
6.2	Right on Graham
6.3	Left on Macon
6.6	Left on Warner
6.9	Right on Iola
7.0	Right on Nanz
7.4	Left on Macon
7.7	Left on Wilmington
8.1	Right on Cannons, left on Trinity
8.4	Right on McCready, left on Trinity
8.5	Spring house
8.7	Left on Beals Branch
9.0	Right on Cannons
9.2	Right on Pee Wee Reese
9.85	Left on Rock Creek
10.0	Back at start

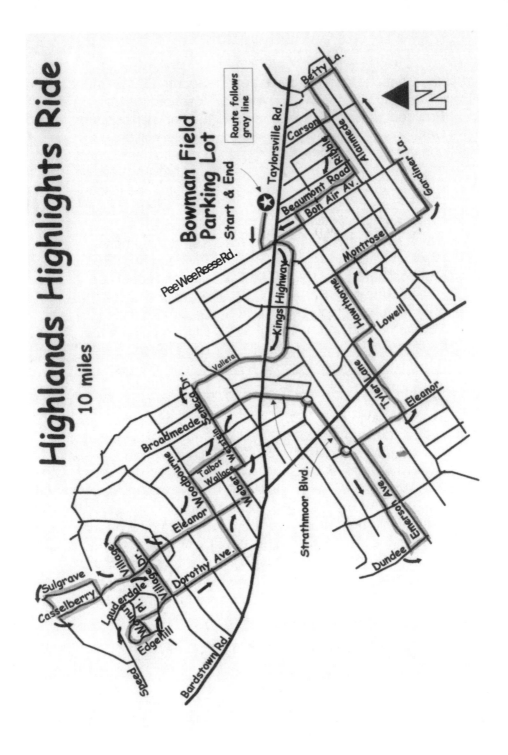

Highlands Highlights Ride

10 miles

Bowman Field Parking Lot
Start & End

Route follows gray line

N

28

Highlands Highlights Ride

Turtle Ride. Ten miles. No hills. Starts at the Bowman Field parking lot, near the corner of Taylorsville Road and Pee Wee Reese Road.

The **Highlands** is a tough place to plot out a Turtle Ride. Turtle Rides can't have hills, and it's hard to find 10 continuous miles through the best of what I call the Highlands, without some pretty good hills. You have to be very careful where you turn, or you will find yourself coasting blissfully downhill, and then you will face an uphill somewhere.

But it is my claim that this ride gets the job done – with some convolutions, to be sure, but only a little bit of overlapping. And maybe one or two minor acclivities that you couldn't really call a hill.

Neighborhoods Galore

I use the term "Highlands" loosely – as I've found a lot of Louisvillians do – to take in a much larger area than that labeled Highlands on neighborhoods maps. Actually, what such maps call the Highlands is what I've always heard called the **"Original Highlands."** This ride doesn't even go there.

I'm talking parts of the area on both sides of the Baxter-Bardstown corridor, from the vicinity of the **Cave Hill Cemetery** entrance to the Watterson Expressway. Actually, if you look on a neighborhoods map, you will find that the ride touches parts of Kingsley, Seneca Gardens, Highlands-Douglas, the Strathmoors (Village, Manor and Gardens), Hayfield Dundee, Gardiner Lane, Wellington and Hawthorne.

Sunday Riding

The core of this ride came from a Sunday outing with my friends Ben and Eileen Hershberg, who like a good ride in a nice neighborhood. Chances are you will see a few fellow cyclists along this route, ranging from toddlers on tricycles to people whose helmets hide gray hair. (Had you thought of that as a reason to cycle?)

Leave the parking lot at **Bowman Field** and turn left onto Pee Wee Reese Road, to take advantage of the traffic light for crossing Taylorsville Road. Then turn right on Kings Highway, and take that delightful street around and back to its intersection with Taylorsville.

29

You'll find yourself on Valetta Road after the crossing, and you'll turn soon on Seneca Drive and then Talbott Avenue to get over to Woodbourne Avenue. There are a lot of great houses all along the way. Before we settled in **Crescent Hill** years ago, my wife, Suzanne, and I used to drive around these streets and dream about living here.

Take Woodbourne down to Eleanor Avenue, turn right, and ride down to Village Drive and take the loop to the right. Take Casselberry Road and turn right again to loop around Sulgrave Road. That's about as far as you can go in that direction without going down a hill.

So hang a left on Cherokee Road and take Casselberry back to Village. Taking a right on Dorothy Avenue lets you go out on another little geographic promontory there, without losing too much altitude if you curl back around on Edgehill Road and Walnut Place.

Lauderdale

Don't go too fast around there, though. There is an **old stone cottage**

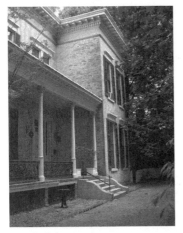

sort of buried in the trees at 2116 Edgehill that was once home to slaves. I was so taken with its stone walls and shake roof the first time I cycled by there that I didn't even notice that there is a huge old mansion even farther back in the trees behind it.

Louisville historian-politician Tom Owen said land records suggest the house is called **Lauderdale**, named by German immigrant Jacob Krieger for his home village, Lautertal. Krieger made money in banking and reared 10 children there.

Lauderdale

Owen said the big house probably was built shortly after the Civil War, on the site of an earlier home owned by William Pope that had burned. He's found records that show the property had a number of owners from Pope to the present.

The slave building is older than the big house, he said, but its age is hard to pin down. It could have been built in the 1820s or so, he said.

That's Louisville

Anyway, those old buildings, tucked away among subdivision houses built in the 1920s, illustrate one of the great things about riding a bike around Louisville. In the Highlands, in Crescent Hill and St. Matthews, everywhere, you're apt to encounter a real relic of the past, still occupied, in the midst of property uses that came along much, much later.

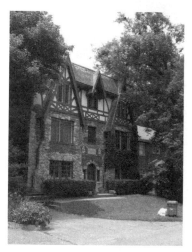

A Highlands apartment building

Take Dorothy Avenue back to Woodbourne, then take Eleanor again and Weber, Wallace and Wetstein avenues. Broadmeade Road will take you back across Taylorsville onto Strathmoor Boulevard, which takes you on across Bardstown Road and up to Dundee Road.

You cut left on Dundee back toward **Atherton High School**, home of the fighting Rebels, and then left again on Emerson Avenue, on a relentless quest to hang on to the level ground. A right on Eleanor and a left on Tyler Lane scoots you back across Bardstown and into Strathmoor Gardens.

A right on Lowell Avenue, a left on Hawthorne Avenue, and a right on Montrose Avenue take you through parts of Hawthorne and Wellington.

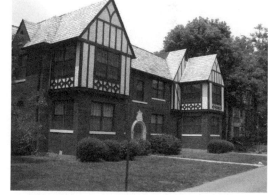

Safety Note: Take care on Montrose. It takes a narrow, pedestrians-and-cyclists-only passage through the trees between Brighton Drive and Alanmede Road. It's easy enough to shoot the gap, but sometimes the drop-off where the pavement ends briefly is a bit abrupt. Don't race through there.

A left on Gardiner Lane takes you along the Watterson Expressway wall, a facility you will no doubt be glad for. The neighborhood you are passing through there and on Betty Lane, Alanmede Road, Carson Way, Ribble Road, and Beaumont Road, has quite a different flavor from, say, the Sulgrave-Casselberry area. It's interesting in its own right.

A left on Hawthorne and a right on Bon Air Avenue takes you back across Taylorsville Road to the start.

Route Sheet

0.0	Leave Bowman Field	4.5	Right on Wallace Avenue and left on Wetstein Avenue
0.1	Left on Pee Wee Reese Road, cross Taylorsville Rd., right on Kings Highway	4.8	Right on Broadmeade Road
		5.0	Cross Taylorsville Road onto Strathmoor Boulevard
0.6	Cross Taylorsville onto Valetta Road	5.2	Around circle, straight on Strathmoor
0.9	Left on Seneca Dr.	5.3	Cross Bardstown
1.22	Right on Talbott Avenue	5.4	Another circle. Straight on Strathmoor
1.4	Left on Woodbourne Avenue	6.1	Left on Dundee Road
1.6	Right on Eleanor Avenue	6.2	Left on Emerson Avenue
1.9	Right on Village Drive	6.0	Right on Eleanor Avenue
2.2	Right on Casselberry Road	7.2	Left on Tyler Lane
2.3	Right on Speed Avenue	7.3	Right on Lowell Avenue
2.4	Left on Sulgrave Road	7.4	Left on Hawthorne Avenue
2.6	Left on Cherokee Road	7.7	Right on Montrose Avenue
2.7	Left on Casselberry Road	8.1	Left on Gardiner Lane
3.1	Right on Village Drive	8.8	Left on Betty Lane
3.3	Right on Dorothy Avenue	8.9	Left on Alanmede Road
3.4	Straight on Edgehill and around	9.1	Right on Carson Way and left on Ribble Road
3.6	Left on Walnut Place	9.2	Right on Beaumont Road
3.7	Right on Dorothy Avenue	9.6	Left on Hawthorne Avenue and right on Bon Air Avenue, cross Taylorsville and turn right
4.1	Left on Woodbourne Avenue		
4.2	Right on Eleanor Avenue		
4.4	Left on Weber Avenue		

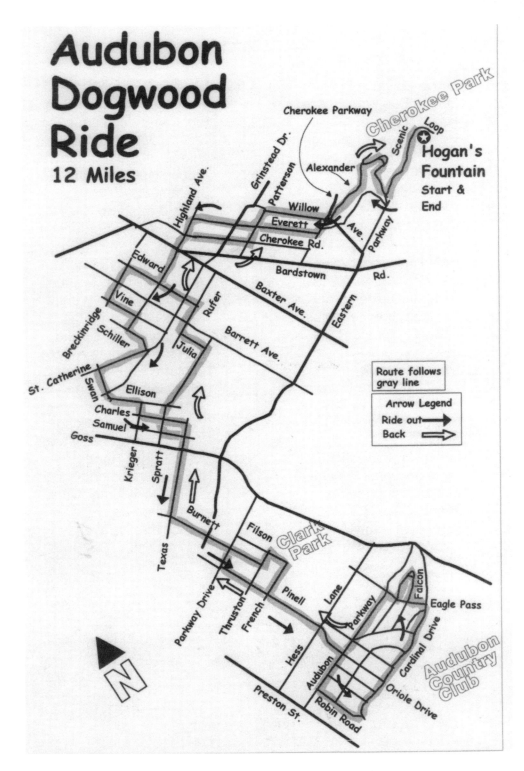

Audubon
Dogwood
Ride
12 Miles

Cherokee Parkway

Cherokee Park

Scenic Loop

Hogan's
Fountain
Start &
End

Alexander

Highland Ave.

Grinstead Dr.

Patterson

Willow

Everett

Cherokee Rd.

Ave.

Parkway

Bardstown

Rd.

Edward

Baxter Ave.

Eastern

Vine

Rufer

Breckinridge

Schiller

Barrett Ave.

Julia

St. Catherine

Swan

Ellison

Route follows
gray line

Charles

Samuel

Arrow Legend

Goss

Ride out

Krieger

Spratt

Back

Burnett

Texas

Filson

Clark
Park

Falcon

Eagle Pass

Parkway Drive

Thruston

Pinell

Lane

Parkway

Cardinal Drive

French

Hess

Audubon

Audubon
Country
Club

Oriole Drive

N

Preston St.

Robin Road

34

Audubon Dogwood Ride

Twelve miles. A few hills, mostly in the park. Start at Hogan's Fountain in Cherokee Park, near the end of Eastern Parkway.

Martha Elson and I worked out this ride one year when we wanted to cycle from our homes in **Crescent Hill** down to **Audubon Park** to see the dogwoods in bloom. The streets are great in Audubon Park about the third week in April, and there's even a festival, with lights and music.

But this ride is good any time of year.

We wanted to get there without going on busy streets such as Eastern Parkway and Poplar Level Road, and maybe to take in some interesting other neighborhoods on the way.

Since most readers don't live at my house or Martha's, I set the start and end at **Hogan's Fountain** in Cherokee Park. There are a couple of hills in the park and it's a little longer than 10 miles. But otherwise, it's a Turtle Ride.

Sallie Bingham

Start out on **Scenic Loop** going down the hill toward Eastern Parkway, taking advantage of city farsightedness that permits cyclists to ride in either the motorist or recreation lane in the park. You're in the recreation lane, so watch out for people with strollers and dog leashes that can suddenly stretch across your path.

Climb back up to Alexander, turn left and enjoy the downhill to the multi-street intersection by the gazebo on Willow Avenue. Be careful of traffic coming in from Willow on your left, and other traffic coming off Cherokee Parkway on both your left and right. When it's safe, climb the little hill on Willow and look at all of the Victorian houses.

The last one on the left before Longest Avenue used to belong to Sallie Bingham, a member of the family that once owned *The Courier-Journal.* It is a marvelous thing to look at. You're in the Cherokee Triangle neighborhood.

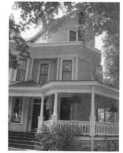

Formerly Sallie Bingham's house

Life in the Triangle

Take a left on Patterson Avenue, and a right on Everett Avenue. There are great old houses all along here.

35

Former *Courier-Journal* reporter Brian Wooley bought a big old house on Everett for a real song – less than $20,000 back in the '70s – and exhausted himself tearing out the old stuff and putting in new.

A couple of partially-inebriated *Courier-Journal* photographers peered in his front window in the wee hours one morning and saw him asleep in a chair in the midst of restoration debris.

They woke him excitedly and told him someone seemed to be stealing the very paper off his walls.

Original Highlands

Cross Grinstead to Highland Avenue, take a left, cross Baxter Avenue and then take a right onto Edward Street. You're in the **Highlands** neighborhood, sometimes called the **Original Highlands** to distinguish it from the much larger area often referred to as the Highlands.

There are picturesque Victorian houses in the Original Highlands, too, and corner taverns.

Turn left on Breckinridge Street and cross Barrett Avenue, which puts you in **Germantown**. Move immediately into the left lane so you can turn left on Vine Street. You make a lot of turns on these neighborhood rides, so you see a lot of streets.

Turn right on Highland Avenue, left on Schiller Avenue, and right on St. Catherine Street. That takes you down to Swan Street, where a left will take you to Ellison Avenue, where you also turn left. Turn right on Krieger Street, left on Charles Street and ride on down to Texas Avenue. A right there will take you across Goss Avenue into Schnitzelburg.

George Rogers Clark's Parents

One doesn't often think of **George Rogers Clark**, hero of the revolution, conqueror of the northwest, founder of Louisville and Clarksville, Indiana, as having parents. But he did, and they moved with several of his siblings to Louisville from Virginia in 1785, after most of the fireworks were over. They're buried just up the route here.

Follow Texas to Burnett Avenue, take a left and cross Eastern Parkway, then take Thruston Avenue left and Filson Avenue right to **George Rogers Clark Park**. Just to the left of the corner where Filson meets French Street, you will see the graves, up among the trees.

John and Ann Rogers Clark were the parents of three generals, including William Clark, a younger brother to George Rogers Clark, who led

Thomas Jefferson's Corp of Discovery with Meriwether Lewis; and Jonathan Clark, an older brother who was a major general in the Virginia Militia.

Several other family members also are buried at the site, which was near **Mulberry Hill**, a large log house that was the Clark home. It was built in 1784 inside what is now the park, and its last remnant was torn down in 1917 after the ground became a part of **Camp Zachary Taylor** in World War I.

The Audubons

Follow French Street away from the park and take a left on Pindell Avenue. You're in the **Audubon** neighborhood, not to be confused with **Audubon Park**, a fifth-class city.

Audubon, the neighborhood, was developed in the 1940s, about 20 years after the most active development of Audubon Park, the city. The neighborhood's houses are much smaller and on smaller lots than most of those in the city, and the *Louisville Encyclopedia* says residents of the city tried to block formation of the neighborhood, because they were afraid it would detract from the unique character of their development.

You enter **Audubon Park** when you cross Hess Lane, where Pindell becomes Oriole Drive. It is quickly apparently that city residents need not have worried. The unique character of their community remains intact, and a marvelous character it is.

Early 20th Century Suburb

Audubon Park was carefully planned by the Audubon Park Realty Co. as a garden suburb, with tree-lined streets and designated green spaces. Most of the houses are big. They are neo-colonial, Dutch-colonial, neo-federal and neo-Tudor, among other things. Some show Spanish influence.

You should really just ride around Audubon Park. It is compact and you can't get lost. Because a bike route has to go somewhere, I took this one left on Audubon Parkway, left on Robin Road, around the historic marker, left on Cardinal Drive at the gates of **Audubon Country Club**.

Then to avoid some, but not all, of the hills, I took it left on Eagle Pass, right into a little loop around Falcon Drive, right on Eagle Pass again, and left on Audubon Parkway.

It's a great long coast on the Parkway back to Oriole Drive, where a right will take you back out of the city, into the neighborhood.

Don't leave too soon just because the route does, though. Anywhere you turn there is something enjoyable to see.

Rivets

Audubon Park is on the glide path for planes going into **Louisville International Airport**, and you may find the occasional plane distracting. Martha and I looked up at one so low you could count the fasteners on its belly.

You follow Oriole onto Pindell and ride up to Parkway Drive, where a right will take you back to Burnett and Texas. After you've crossed Goss Avenue, take Samuel Street left instead of Charles, just to see another Germantown street, and then take Spratt Street down to Ellison Avenue.

Take Ellison right rather than following it back the way you came. Get over to the left side of Ellison and climb the little hill onto Julia Avenue. A right on Rufer Avenue and a careful crossing of Barrett will take you to a left on Edward and a right on Highland.

Back to the Start

Take Cherokee Road this time, back as far as Patterson, and then turn left, go to Everett and follow it down to Cherokee Parkway. Go left and stay straight down to Willow—taking the parkway fork that goes left of the gazebo—and negotiate the crossing onto Alexander and up into **Cherokee Park**.

Scenic Loop takes you back to **Hogan's Fountain**, traveling in the traffic lane this time.

Map Matters

This is one of two maps in the book that I found I could get a little larger within the page size if I tilted it so that north is some direction other than straight up. The other one is the Mitchell Hill Ride. They are both vaguely kidney-shaped, interestingly.

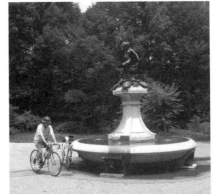

Ben Hershberg at Hogan's Fountain

Route Sheet

0.0	Leave Hogan's Fountain parking lot on Scenic Loop	5.6	Right on Audubon Parkway
0.9	Left on Alexander	5.9	Left around historic marker on Robin Road
1.3	Cross Cherokee Parkway and go straight on Willow Avenue.	6.2	Left on Cardinal Drive at gates to country club
1.6	Left on Patterson Avenue, right on Everett Ave.	6.9	Left on Eagle Pass
1.7	Cross Grinstead Drive	6.0	Right on Falcon Drive, and follow around to left
2.0	Left on Highland Avenue	6.4	Right on Eagle Pass and left on Audubon Parkway
2.1	Cross Baxter		
2.3	Right on Edward Street	6.8	Right on Oriole Drive
2.5	Left on Breckinridge, cross Barrett, moving to the left lane	7.6	Right on Parkway Drive
		7.7	Left on Burnett Avenue
		8.1	Right on Texas Avenue
2.6	Left on Vine Street	8.5	Left on Samuel Street
2.8	Right on Highland Avenue	8.7	Right on Spratt Street
2.9	Left on Schiller Avenue	8.8	Right on Ellison Avenue
3.0	Right on St. Catherine Street	9.1	Left on Julia Avenue
		9.2	Right on Rufer Avenue
3.3	Left on Swan	9.3	Left on Edward Street
3.4	Left on Ellison Avenue	9.5	Right on Highland Avenue
3.5	Right on Krieger Street	9.8	Right on Cherokee Road
3.6	Left on Charles Street	10.1	Left on Patterson Avenue
3.9	Right on Texas Avenue	10.2	Right on Everett Avenue
4.4	Left on Burnett Avenue	10.5	Left on Cherokee Parkway
4.8	Left on Thruston Avenue	10.6	Cross Willow Avenue, straight on Alexander
4.9	Right on Filson Avenue		
5.0	Right on French Street	11.0	Right on Scenic Loop
5.2	Left on Pindell Avenue	11.8	Back at parking lot
5.5	Cross Hess Lane, bear right on Oriole Drive		

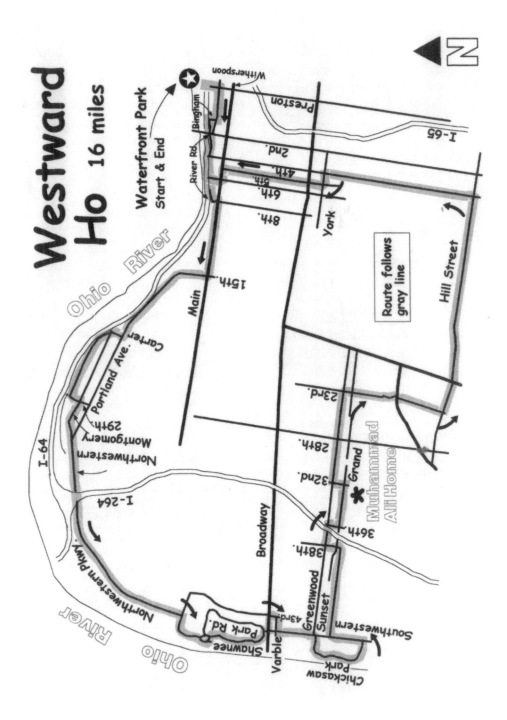

Westward Ho 16 miles

Waterfront Park
Start & End

Route follows gray line

Westward Ho

Sixteen miles. Almost flat. Start at Waterfront Park, off River Road, near Preston Street.

Back in 1984, I planned a bike route for a *Louisville Times* Neighborhoods ride that took in part of the **West End**, an area that has had mostly black residents since the 1960s. It was a real eye-opener for some people – especially white people, who hadn't ventured into that part of town for years, if ever.

White flight in civil rights days, a full-fledged riot in the Parkland neighborhood in 1968, and some nasty brick-throwing incidents that shut down the popular **Fontaine Ferry Park** in 1969, caused a lot of people to write the West End off.

I think a lot of those white riders expected serious slums, if not burned-out hulks, to predominate. Consequently, they marveled at the old mansions and tidy cottages that are everywhere in that part of town.

Many of the neighborhoods have improved a lot even since that ride, with landmark housing projects, and envelope-pushing commercial developments leading the way. Now efforts are underway to reclaim some of the "brown fields" industrial sites that dot the area, to provide more jobs and bring the West End back up to its potential.

It's a good time to check the place out.

Potential Combo

This ride is about half of the 1984 *Times* Neighborhoods ride, modified a bit in the West End to pass such landmarks as **Muhammad Ali's boyhood home**. If you're up for more than a 16-mile outing, try combining it with the downtown-to-Crescent Hill "Near East" ride that's next in the book. That will make it 30 – or 23 if you

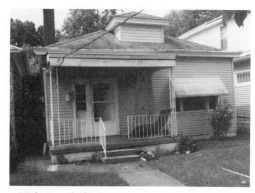

Muhammad Ali's home

take a shortcut I point out. The two rides originally were part of the same ride, though riders were given shortcut options then, too.

Take Your Choice

And speaking of choices, this ride offers you either a marvelous ride along the **Louisville RiverWalk**, or a quite scintillating tour of part of West Main Street and of the old turnpike along which freight wagons hauled tons of goods around the falls of the Ohio, before the Portland Canal was built in 1830.

To take either, you turn right out of the of the park and take a couple of more rights onto Witherspoon and Bingham Way, then follow River Road until it reaches Eighth Street.

Safety Note: There's a traffic light at Third and River Road, where traffic comes down off I-64. When you have the traffic light on River Road, traffic going straight on Third Street is stopped. But traffic turning right off the ramp onto River Road is permitted to go at any time.

So, as you proceed through the light and make your way to the right side of River Road after the intersection, watch out for cars barreling down the ramp and making a right turn right into the place where you are.

Eighth Street brings decision time. You can cut right through the parking lot and onto the **RiverWalk**. Or you can go left up a slight hill to a right turn onto Main Street.

It's a great ride either way, but you should be aware that the RiverWalk is sometimes blocked by mud during high water times, and you may find yourself backtracking.

Whether you take the RiverWalk or Main Street the first time you do this ride, I recommend you take the other the next time. And alternate from then on, season permitting, until you're just too old to do it anymore. People have been known to cycle well into their 90s, though.

Safety Note: Bikeways are controversial among experienced cyclists, because they can create hazards while giving an illusion of safety. Studies show that cyclists are actually more likely to collide with motor traffic where bike paths intersect with streets than they would be if they just stayed on the street.

The designers of the RiverWalk have created a path with very few intersections, though, and it is by and large a joy to ride. But be aware that cyclists share it with strollers, skaters, baby buggies and other pedestrians.

In some ways, bikes are less compatible with pedestrian traffic than they are with automotive traffic. Like cars, bikes tend to go along in fairly straight, predictable lines. Pedestrians, on the other hand, can change course instantly, in any direction, with no notice. So be careful, for your sake and theirs. Slow down when you are around them.

Premier Path

That said, it should be noted that the RiverWalk is a great place to ride. It is refreshing to be away from motor traffic, and there are great views of the **Portland Canal** and the river all along it.

There are mileage markers embedded in the pavement, along with information on river lore. The level of Louisville's record 1937 flood is marked in several places.

You can pop off the path near 23rd Street to see the **Portland Museum** if you like. More about that later. Backtrack to the path, and follow its markings on around through some woods to **Shawnee Park.**

When the route drops down off the floodwall in the vicinity of **Shawnee Golf Course**, it meanders through a grove of gnarled old cottonwood trees that always reminds me of the forest in the Wizard of Oz. The walk emerges at the **Olmsted-designed Lily Pond in Shawnee Park,** where you can rejoin the street portion of the ride.

Big Baseball Bat

On those times when you don't take the RiverWalk, turn left on Eighth Street and climb the hill onto Main. You get a short stretch of the cast iron building fronts and restored splendor of historic West Main.

Stay to the right there, but notice the **Hillerich & Bradsby baseball bat** on the left, appearing to lean against the building. It's the world's largest – 120 feet long, with a barrel 9 feet in diameter and weighing in at 68,000 pounds. It marks the entrance of the **Louisville Slugger** maker's bat museum, and the actual factory where the company still turns out bats for major leaguers.

Great tours are offered. There's a 21-ton limestone glove inside. That big bat's made of steel, but it will look remarkably like wood from your vantage point across the street.

Don't overlook the companion baseball smashing through a dummy window high on another building a little farther down the street.

Roadside Brigands

Stay on Main Street until 15th Street, then turn right and wind down past the old **B & O (for Baltimore and Ohio) railroad freight station**. The street goes left after that and becomes Portland Avenue, which follows the route of an old turnpike where wagons once rumbled along with goods being portaged around the falls of the Ohio. The need to portage is the reason Louisville is here.

The **Portland Canal**, built in 1830, permitted boats to bypass the falls without unloading. But before that, bandits used to lie in wait along the turnpike to sample the rich cargo. They've long since been run off by Portland residents, though.

Stay on Portland Avenue through the Portland neighborhood, which has remained a white enclave in mostly black West Louisville. Portland was a city in its own right, twice, before it was annexed to Louisville for the final time in 1852.

It was a home of river captains, and of the 7-feet-8-inches-tall **"Kentucky Giant" Jim Porter**, who had taverns there and in **Shippingport**, a town on Shippingport Island that was wiped out by floods and canal building.

Succor for Seamen

Turn right off Portland onto Carter Street. There are two landmarks there. On your right, the **Unique Thrift Store**, which offers great bargains. I once bought an almost new pair of wool slacks there for $2 and had them made into knickers, which are still my favorite way to go for winter riding.

On the left is the old **U.S. Marine Hospital**, built by the state and opened in 1847 as a place to treat merchant seamen from boats passing through the canal. A larger building erected to replace the old hospital is now the **Portland Family Health Center**.

If you've got a little time for an educational detour, you'll find the **Portland Museum** at 2308 Portland Avenue between 23rd and 24th Streets. It has a lot of river history, and is the heart of the Portland Historic District.

It's open from 10 a.m. to 4:30 p.m. Tuesday through Friday. It costs $5 for adults and $4 for children over six and seniors, and it's free for everybody on Wednesdays.

Backtrack to Northwestern Parkway. At 29th Street you can take another detour to follow the River Walk up over the floodwall and visit **Wharf Park**, a restoration project that is underway on the flat ground beyond the K&I Bridge. It could be muddy in the wrong season, though.

Buy Stuff

You will note a number of eateries all along this ride, many of them intriguing. Some offer beer. Explore and enjoy. But be sure your bike is secure, and don't hurt yourself.

Shawnee Surprise

Take 29th Street to Montgomery Street, turn right, and you'll soon find yourself cruising along Northwestern Parkway. It was along this stretch on the 1984 *Louisville Times* ride when I started hearing oohs and ahhs from people who didn't expect to find attractive real estate.

It's a parkway, and there are nice houses along it, in some pretty diverse styles, ranging from Tudor to Italianate, Renaissance Revival and Victorian Gothic.

On the right, you'll pass the **Shawnee Golf Course**, which for some time also was a fairly well-kept secret. When William Stansbury was mayor of Louisville from 1977 to 1981, he took a lot of heat from the press. A story went around that he used to hang out at the Shawnee course because it was a place no reporters would ever find him.

Fontaine Ferry Park

Further along on the right, you'll pass the now-leveled site of **Fontaine Ferry Park** – better known as Fountain Ferry, dear to the memory of many a white Louisville native, but tainted with segregation issues for many blacks. It was a popular summer picnic spot, with a large swimming pool with a waterfall, a succession of spectacular roller coasters and other rides, and the Gypsy Village dance garden.

Internationally known bicycle racers set world records on Fontaine Ferry's one-third-mile velodrome during the 1896 meet of the League of American Wheelmen – a national cycling organization that was then at the height of political power and social popularity.

Turn right onto Shawnee Park Road and enter the broad park that designer **Frederick Law Olmsted** supposed would be a great place for lawn games. It has many playing fields today.

Tobacco Mansion
Olmsted's Lily Pond, where the RiverWalk leaves the river and takes to city sidewalks, is on the south end of the park. Pass it and proceed out onto Broadway and turn left for a look at **Basil Doerhoefer's mansion**, at 4432 W. Broadway.

Doerhoefer was a tobacco manufacturing executive who owned a lot of land in the vicinity before the park was laid out. His family had other mansions in the Shawnee neighborhood. His mansion later served as **Loretto High School** – a Catholic girls' school – for many years and now is owned by Christ Temple Apostolic Church.

Segregation
Go South on 44th Street then and turn right onto Varble Avenue to get back to Southwestern Parkway. Turn left and follow it down to **Chickasaw Park.**

Chickasaw is a beautiful park with the distinction of being the only city park black people could use until Mayor Andrew Broadus ordered all parks, swimming pools and amphitheaters to admit all races in 1955.

Chickasaw was established in 1922 on the estate of John "Boss" Whallen, a Democratic power broker.

A Black Architect
Head back up Southwestern Parkway out of Chickasaw, and turn right on Sunset Avenue. The first street you pass – it will be on the right – is **Plato Terrace**, named for Samuel Plato, a black architect who Louisville historian Walter Hutchins says designed and built many of the houses in the area you are passing through.

Plato learned architecture and carpentry through a correspondence school, and ultimately developed his expertise enough to land the contracts for 40 or more U.S. post offices around the country. He also designed the Classical Revival **Broadway Temple A.M.E. Church** at 15th and Broadway, among other buildings in the West End.

Home of The Greatest

There are a number of impediments to straight-through streets in this part of town, and it takes a little wandering to get onto **Muhammad Ali's** section of Grand Avenue. Go left at 38th Street, right on Greenwood Avenue, right on 36th Street, and left on Grand.

The unprepossessing house at 3302 Grand Ave. is where the three-time heavyweight boxing champion, and international humanitarian, grew up. He was **Cassius Marcellus Clay** in those days.

Once when I was riding by the house, I talked with J.C. Stephenson, who said he and his father, Steve, had bought it four years previously as rental property.

When they bought it, he said, they didn't know who had lived there. In the process of getting it ready for tenants, J.C. said he found a box of junk up in the attic that included one boxing glove.

He said he looked all around for the mate, but didn't find it, so he threw the first one away with the other junk. Later, a neighbor told him whose house it had been. "When I found out, that glove was the first thing that came to my mind," he said. But it was long gone by then.

1968 Riot

Turn left on 32nd Street and take Greenwood again. You're riding through the **Parkland neighborhood**, another section of town that was a city in its own right until it was annexed by Louisville in 1894.

The section along 28th Street in the vicinity of Dumesnil St. and Greenwood was a thriving commercial center until May, 1968. Then rioting, amidst tension that followed the assassination of Dr. Martin Luther King in Memphis, shattered many businesses and drove their owners out of the area.

The unrest broke out at 28th and Greenwood. Before it was over two teenagers had been killed—one by police and another by a liquor store owner—and much property damaged.

Cabbage Patch

Stay on Greenwood to 23rd Street, then turn right opposite **Victory Park**, and head down to Hill Street. It will take a couple of jogs, at Dumesnil and Wilson Streets.

The area along Hill Street between 14th and 7th streets is mostly industrial now, but it once was a sort of ramshackle neighborhood along the railroad tracks, made famous by Alice Hegan Rice's 1901 novel, *Mrs. Wiggs of the Cabbage Patch.*

Historic Fourth Street

Turn left at Fourth Street and head downtown, noting the many 19th century mansions on the way. That's **Central Park** on the left after Magnolia Street, site of a huge international exposition in the 1880s.

At Fourth and Kentucky you pass **Memorial Coliseum**, venue for a sufficient number of big name entertainers since 1929 that it rates a historical marker. On those front steps, in 1952, fiery Louisville labor leader Pat Ansbury danced a jig when he heard that Adlai Stevenson was the Democratic nominee for the presidency, and collapsed and died.

Across the street is **Memorial Park**, where you can rest on replicas of Grecian ruins, or on a bench covered with mosaic art created mostly by students. Contemplate the distinctive tree sculpture.

You'll pass through **Spalding University** as you approach York Street. The building that houses the **Spalding University Center** on the left just before you reach the **800 apartment building** – near York Street – was once the **Columbia Gymnasium**. There, Louisville policeman Joe Martin taught a young Cassius Clay how to box, in the 1950s.

Turn left onto York Street, then right onto Fifth.

Fifth Street

That big church on the right just past Muhammad Ali Boulevard is the **Catholic Cathedral of the Assumption,** built between 1849 and 1852. The **Jefferson County Court House**, on the left after you pass Jefferson Street, was designed by Kentucky architect **Gideon Shryock.** Problems stretched its construction out from 1836 to 1860.

Take a left onto Main Street. That's the postmodern **Humana Building** on the left, built between 1982 and 1985, and the **Kentucky Center for the Arts** on the right. The arts center opened in 1983 and has presented Kentuckians with classical performing arts programs and Broadway shows.

Turn right on Sixth Street and follow River Road, Bingham and Witherspoon back to the Park. Depending on the season, you will likely see the steamboat **Belle of Louisville**, the pseudo steamboat **Spirit of Jefferson**, and the **Star of Louisville dinner boat** along the wharf there. And you may even see the huge **American Queen** steamboat.

Route Sheet

0.0	Right on River Road from park	9.4	Right on Greenwood
0.2	Right on Witherspoon	9.6	Right on 36th
0.5	Right on Bingham becomes River Road	9.7	Left on Grand
		9.9	3302 Grand, Muhammed Ali home
1.3	Left on 8th, right on Main	10.0	Left on 32nd.
1.8	Right on 15th bears left, becomes Portland Ave.	10.1	Right on Greenwood
2.8	Right on Carter, left on Northwestern Parkway	10.4	28th and Greenwood - riot center
		10.8	Right on 23rd.
3.6	The Java House	11.1	Jog left, then right at Dumesnil
3.7	Left on 29th St.		
3.8	Right on Montgomery	11.2	Jog right, then left at Wilson
4.0	It becomes Northwestern	11.7	Left on Hill
5.1	Pass golf course club house	12.5	or so Cabbage Patch
6.0	Right into Shawnee Park	13.0	Left on Fourth
6.4	Bear right, then left, then right	13.9	Memorial Park on right Memorial Colliseum on left
6.8	Lily Pond		
7.0	Left onto Broadway	14.2	Former Columbia Gym, left on York
7.1	Right onto 45th Street and right onto Varble Avenue		
		14.3	Right on Fifth
7.2	Left onto Southwestern	15.2	Left on Main
7.6	Right into Chickasaw Park	15.3	Right on Sixth
8.2	Left onto Southwestern	15.4	Right on River Road
8.5	Right onto Sunset	15.9	Left on Witherspoon
9.2	Left onto 38th St.	16.3	Left on River Road
		16.4	Finish at park

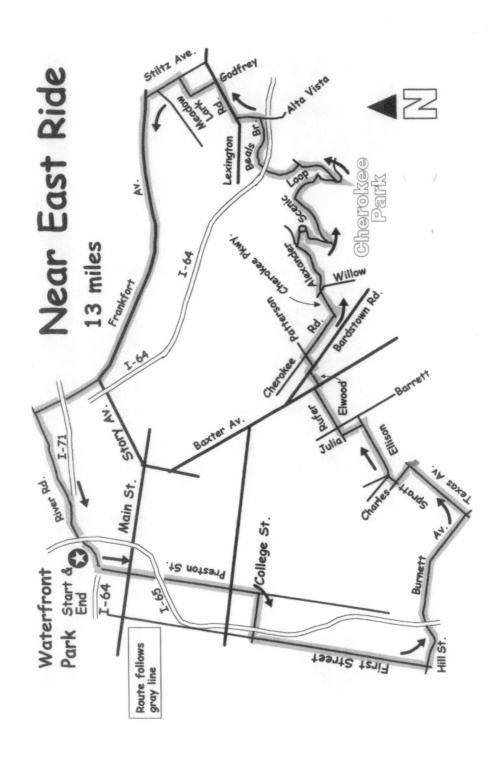

Near East Ride
13 miles

Waterfront Park
Start & End

Route follows gray line

N

50

Near East Ride

Thirteen miles. A few hills, but no big ones. Potential for traffic. Start at Waterfront Park, off River Road, near Preston Street.

This ride is basically the eastern half of the 1984 *Louisville Times* Neighborhoods ride, for which I laid out the route as the newspaper company's resident cycling fanatic. I separated it from the western half for this book—see Westward Ho, the ride just before this one—to make each a little easier to accomplish. The halves can be put back together, though. And I recommend that if you have enough time, or have worked your way up to longer rides.

To recombine, you could just stay on Hill Street as you come east from the West End and keep on going out through Germantown. Or you could loop downtown and back out to Hill so as not to miss the good stuff downtown and in Old Louisville. The combined ride is almost 30 miles if you don't take a shortcut on Hill Street. It's a little over 23 if you do.

Cruising the Nabes

The original ride was intended to promote the late great *Times'* Neighborhoods section, which was fairly new then. The thought was that Louisville might be a more cohesive place if readers saw each others' neighborhoods in more detail than you get just passing through in a car. So we strung together as many neighborhoods as we thought we could without killing the riders off.

As it was, we set the thing up so the rider could complete the west end portion and then just head back to the starting point at the Belvedere if he'd had enough. Or, he could stay the course and do the whole ride. Many took the short cut. Others went on, but found their own short cuts back to the starting place as they wore out.

Some people just couldn't get past inviting landmarks along the way. I believe we lost a bunch of people – including then-mayor Harvey Sloane and a couple of his kids, who were young then – either at **Heitzman's Bakery** in Germantown, or cater-corner across the street at **Check's Café**. Heitzman's, alas, moved from that building in the summer of 2002.

Exotic Architecture

Head out of the Park and up Preston Street. You're in part of Mayor David Armstrong's "**e-Main**" revitalization district, and you will see major projects in both new and very old buildings in this part of town.

Stay to the right all the way up past Broadway, then turn onto College Street, and zip under the Interstate for a left turn onto First.

That domed building on the right at Brook Street is **Unity Temple**, a multi-denominational Christian Church. When it was built in 1919, though, it was the home of the **Adath Jeshuran** Jewish congregation, which now has a building on Woodbourne Avenue.

Victorian Treasure

Passing through a zone of commercial and industrial buildings, you soon find yourself in **Old Louisville**, with Victorian mansions lining both sides of the street.

When I came to Louisville from Montana in 1968, I couldn't believe my eyes in Old Louisville. There were so many brick mansions, street after street of them. Some could be bought then for $11,000 or $12,000. You needed to bring a lot of elbow grease and a wheelbarrow of additional cash to make them livable, and keep them stable, but a lot of people did it.

What I didn't know then is that this is the heart of Victorian America – with a larger concentration of Victorian houses than in any other city in the country. Louisville snoozed while urban renewal took such houses in many cities, and then woke up in time to save its own.

A Place for Holidays

Some of these houses are open for tours at Christmastime, and it's easy to imagine you're in a Currier & Ives print, or expecting a visit from St. Nick at any time. The Old Louisville web site conjures up prominent Louisville families, dressed in their Easter finery, making their way down these streets to the various churches in the spring of 1887. "You can almost hear an orchestra playing 'Easter Parade,'" it says. Indeed.

The heyday of this area was between 1870 and the early 1900s, and it went into serious decline in the 1940s, '50s and '60s. Many of the houses were cut up for apartments and rooming houses. The area has been on the upswing since the late '60s, and many prominent Louisvillians live there again now.

Watch along the route for shops, groceries, bars and eateries, which are numerous and mostly charming.

Germantown

As Hill Street passes Brook Street, you begin to see why this route wasn't on the earlier Nabes Turtle Ride. You roll down into an underpass, then bear left through the light, and then climb out of the underpass.

Safety Note: You'll build up a little speed going down into the Hill Street underpass, and make a slight turn. There's a stoplight at the bottom, and you can't tell whether it's red or green until you're well down the hill. Be careful. Also, as the street becomes Burnett Avenue on the other side of the underpass, traffic rules require that you be in the left lane to go straight. Watch for other traffic jockeying to get into one lane or the other for the intersection at the top of the hill.

Once out of the underpass and straightened out on Burnett, you'll pass into the Germantown neighborhood, and by one of its treasures – the aforementioned **Check's Café**. Feel free to stop for a snack, or for lunch. Be careful where you leave the bikes, though. Lock them, find a place to get them out of sight, or have one person watch them.

Check's is open from 11 a.m. to 10 p.m. Monday through Thursday, and 11 a.m. to 1 a.m. Friday and Saturday. It's open from 1 p.m. to 10 p.m. on Sundays.

Around the Cemetery

Turn on Texas Avenue and proceed down toward **St. Michael Cemetery**. The Nabes ride earlier in this book goes right through the cemetery, with its aging German-language tombstones, and that is a great thing to do.

Sometimes the cemetery is closed, though, so this ride shows you how to get around it. You take a left onto Charles Street and a right onto Spratt Street, then another right onto Ellison Avenue at a multi-street intersection.

On up Ellison, you'll need to get into the left side of the lane when you've passed the cemetery, because you'll want to turn left onto Julia Avevue, a small street. You might want to gear down, too, because Julia takes a sort of a sharp little climb there.

Tyler Park

Zip up over Julia and down the other side to Rufer Avenue, hang a right and go on across Barrett Avenue. You'll pass through a sliver of the Tyler Park neighborhood there, on a course soon to take you into the **Cherokee Triangle.**

There are a couple of right-left jogs in there that can be a little tricky, depending on the time of day. First you turn right onto Baxter Avenue from Rufer Avenue, and left almost immediately onto Ellwood Avenue.

That takes you up to Bardstown Road, where you do the same thing to get across onto Patterson Avenue.

Safety Note: The trick in right-left jogs across busy streets is to wait for the traffic to clear from the left, then move right out into the left side of the center lane, ready to turn left.

When there's a gap in oncoming traffic, complete the turn. It's a piece o' cake, really, but it does require paying attention. It might, in fact, cause you not to notice La Peche there on the corner—one of Bardstown Road's famous eateries, and not a bad place to get a sandwich.

Cherokee Road

After a short stretch on Patterson, you turn right onto Cherokee Road, and you're back in Victorian splendor. The big houses along there were built mostly starting in the 1880s, just a step behind those in Old Louisville.

There wasn't much public transportation out in this direction in the early days of its development, so the first people to build here were wealthy enough to have their own vehicles. The triangle started to decline after World War II, and many mansions became apartment buildings.

Countermeasures started mostly in the early 1960s.

Meet the General

Bear right around the circle when you arrive at Cherokee Parkway, then crank around to the left on the far side of **Gen. John Breckinridge**

Castleman, who is cast in bronze there on his horse, Caroline. They say she posed for the sculptor along with him.

Castleman was a confederate major in the Civil War and he became a federal general in the Spanish American War. He also served on Louisville's Board of Park Commissioners for more than 25 years, and was instrumental in development of the city's parks.

As a cyclist, you will want to know that he was the city's official hospitality host in 1896 when thousands of cyclists from all over the country came to Louisville for the League of American Wheelmen convention. Still, they cast him here on a horse.

Cherokee Park

Proceed down Cherokee Parkway to its intersection with Willow Avenue, look for an opening and zip across onto Alexander and up the hill into Cherokee Park.

You get a taste there of some of the fine work of Castleman's parks board. Turn right onto **Scenic Loop** and catch the view down across the meadow. The slope there often is called **"Dog Hill"** because it has been a popular spot for dog owners to let their animals run.

Roll on down the hill, and back up to the left, to **Hogan's Fountain**. That's the Greek God "Pan" atop the fountain, which was originally a watering fixture for dogs and horses. It was erected in 1903 with money donated by Mr. and Mrs. W.J. Hogan of Anchorage.

With the shelter house on the right and the restrooms and playing fields nearby, the fountain area has been a popular picnic and gathering place for decades. It's a good place to start and end bike rides.

Crossing the Park

You follow the loop down from Hogan's Fountain. It makes a left turn there, onto a section of road that has long been known as **Lover's Lane**, though the signs now call it **Scenic Loop**.

It's a popular walking place. Follow it to the bridge, then bear left and along the grassy flats. In times past, it was possible to catch the occasional whiff of pot smoke on this stretch on a balmy spring day. Take a right onto Beals Branch Road, under I-64 and up the hill to Alta Vista Road.

You've just traversed one of only about three routes that bisect Cherokee Park – which is really just a long skinny place along **Beargrass Creek**, but which is deceptive because of its hills and the curves in its roads.

I know people who just sort of plunge into the park on one side without really knowing where they'll come out on the other. Once you ride around the park a few times on a bicycle, though, it all becomes clear.

Baptist Seminary

As you climb Beals Branch into a left turn onto Alta Vista, you'll pass the elegant residence of the president of the **Southern Baptist Theological**

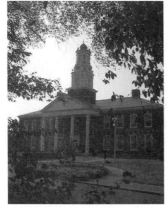

Seminary. If you can get a glimpse through the trees on the right side of Alta Vista Road, you'll see there are similar mansions back from the street, but they now have other large houses in their front yards.

Turn right onto Lexington Road, and you find yourself traveling along the front of the seminary itself. It dates from the 1920s and has had many celebrated professors, though a large number of faculty members left after a sharp turn to the conservative by the seminary's board in the early 1990s.

Southern Baptist Theological Seminary

Get over to the left side of the inside lane there as you pass the last of the seminary buildings – being careful of traffic, of course – so you can turn left onto Godfrey.

Crescent Hill

You're in Crescent Hill now, said to be named for a long, now hardly perceptible, crescent curve in the ridge up Frankfort Avenue toward the **Louisville Water Co.** property you'll soon see on your right at Stiltz Avenue and Frankfort Avenue.

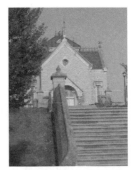

First though, you'll go through a cozy little neighborhood tucked in between the seminary and Stiltz, one long occupied by people connected in one way or another with the seminary. Stay on Godfrey down to Meadowlark Avenue. Turn right, then turn left again on Stiltz.

Louisville Water Company building at the Crescent Hill Reservoir

As you climb up to Frankfort Avenue, you'll pass a stone retaining structure known in the area as the **Chinese Wall**. It is part of Louisville Water Co. facilities more than a century old, where lessons were learned in filtering silt-laden river water that were later put to use in many cities across the country.

Historic Frankfort Avenue

Turn left on Frankfort and you'll cycle a good part of the length of Frankfort Avenue, a street that became trendy in the 1990s. Restaurants, coffee shops, antique stores and the like have proliferated, drawing sport utility vehicles and other upscale transportation.

It's still pretty civilized for cycling, but it's a good idea to be aware of any traffic buildup behind you, and to make an extra effort occasionally to let it by.

After you cross the railroad tracks, be sure to notice the venerable grounds of the **American Printing House for the Blind,** which is the largest publishing house for the visually impaired in the world. Along with books in Braille and large type, it produces talking books and other materials needed by blind people for education and life. I recommend the **Callahan Museum** inside.

Its first building was erected in 1883. Next door is the **Kentucky School for the Blind,** which dates to the 1850s at this site.

Future Greatness

On down Frankfort, you pass Mellwood and Story avenues, and move onto an industrial stretch of Frankfort that has a brighter future if the Frankfort Avenue Business Association gets its way. That stretch used to be called Ohio Street. The association got the name changed as part of general efforts to improve Frankfort Avenue's image.

Jim Goodwin, who has been active in the group, said activity was picking up at restaurants and other businesses along the street, but it was hard to tell visitors how to get there from downtown.

With the name change, Goodwin said, "You could just say, 'Go out River Road and turn right on Frankfort.'"

The future of that stretch is likely to be altered by the reconstruction of Spaghetti Junction, where all of the interstate highways come together downtown, and Goodwin said an extension of Witherspoon Street from the baseball park could reach Frankfort.

Alderwoman Tina Ward-Pugh said there has been talk of a signature entrance for Frankfort Avenue at River Road some day.

Biking Across the Ohio

Turn left on River Road and ride through the developing **Waterfront Park** additions. The plan is that, some day, you'll be able to cycle right up a spiraling path to the end of the **Big Four Bridge**, first opened in 1895 and rebuilt in 1928, and across the river to Jeffersonville, Indiana.

Meanwhile, though, return to your start at Waterfront Park.

Route Sheet

0.0	Right onto River Road from Waterfront Park
0.2	Straight on Preston
1.3	Right on College
1.6	Left on First
2.1	Ermin's Bakery
2.8	Left on Hill
3.8	Checks
3.9	Left on Texas
4.5	Left on Charles
4.6	Right on Spratt
4.7	Right on Ellison
5.0	Left on Julia
5.2	Right on Rufer
5.6	Right on Baxter, left on Elwood
5.7	Right on Bardstown, left on Patterson
5.9	Right on Cherokee Road
6.2	Left on Cherokee Parkway
6.4	Cross Willow. enter Park on Alexander
6.8	Right on Scenic Loop
7.9	Left on Lovers Lane
8.3	Right on Beals Branch
8.8	Left on Alta Vista
9.0	Right on Lexington
9.2	Left on Godfrey
9.4	Right on Meadowlark
9.6	Left on Stiltz
9.9	Left on Frankfort
12.3	Left on River Road
13.4	Right into Park

Locust Grove Ride
19 miles

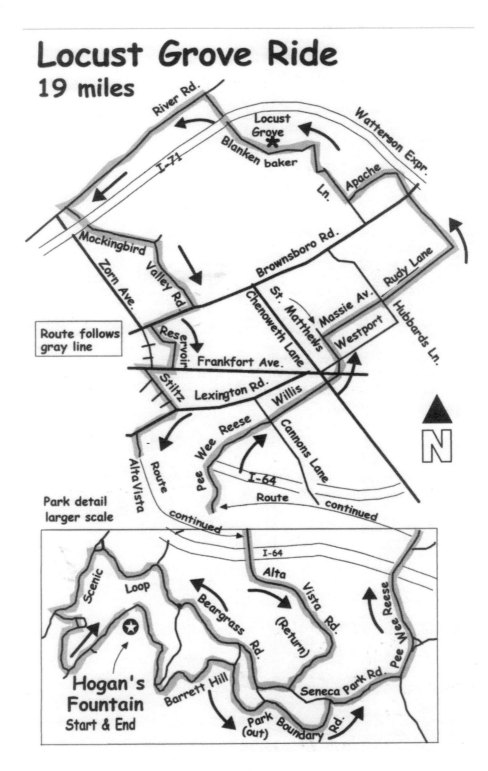

Route follows gray line

Park detail larger scale

Hogan's Fountain
Start & End

Locust Grove Ride

Nineteen miles. Some moderate-to-difficult hills. Potential for traffic in places. Start at Hogan's Fountain, on Scenic Loop in Cherokee Park, just up from the end of Eastern Parkway.

This is a traditional Louisville Bicycle Club ride, meant to let cyclists get a few more miles than they would by just riding around the park. It takes in a good chunk of the rolling freshness of **Cherokee Park**, one of Louisville's three original Olmsted Parks.

A ride in Cherokee involves a few hills, and this ride includes the toughest. I've long maintained that if you practice enough in the park, you'll get all the conditioning you need to ride anywhere.

It starts off with a nice downhill, off the **Hogan's Fountain** hill, and then a significant climb up toward **Chauffeur's Rest**, and continues on in that manner, pretty much up and down, until you top the last park hill to cross Interstate 64 and cruise along the **Seneca Park** playing fields.

St. Matthews

A straight shot up Willis Avenue takes you to the heart of **St. Matthews**, and lets you cross Shelbyville Road at a traffic light, straight ahead onto St. Matthews Avenue.

Safety Note: You jog right and then left to get across Westport Road and the CSX railroad tracks, and there is sometimes a lot of traffic there. There's a stop sign on the left to protect your rear from traffic once you're out on Westport Road, but you have to watch for oncoming traffic so you can make that left turn. Take care.

Massie Avenue and Rudy Lane

You get a nice long straight stretch through a pleasant St. Matthews neighborhood and into **Windy Hills** along Massie Avenue and Rudy Lane. It's interrupted only by another jog right and left at Hubbards Lane. Hubbards traffic is not impeded by traffic signals, so you have to watch your front and your back on that jog.

Rudy Lane takes you around to the left and up to a traffic light at Brownsboro Road, where you can zip across into the friendlier streets of the **Winding Falls** and **Indian Hills-Cherokee** communities.

Zachary Taylor

Hang a left on Apache Road and you'll soon come up on **Springfield**, the boyhood home of **Zachary Taylor** — a.k.a. "Old Rough and Ready." It's a Georgian-style brick mansion completed in the 1780s. Taylor was a Mexican War general who became the twelfth U.S. president in 1849, and

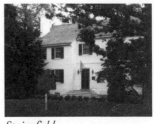

Springfield

died in 1850. He's buried not far from Springfield in a national cemetery named for him.

A theory that Taylor had been poisoned gained such credibility in 1991 that officials took his body out of its tomb to check it out. But the examination was inconclusive.

Among other things, Taylor was father-in-law to Jefferson Davis, president of the Confederacy. His house is one of the few presidential homes in the country that is in private hands. It once belonged to the late *Courier-Journal* columnist Hugh Haynie, who spent a lot of money on it, and who reportedly occasionally threw a lively party there.

George Rogers Clark

Take a right at Blankenbaker Lane and proceed down the hill, up another hill and around to the right to **Locust Grove**. Traffic has picked up

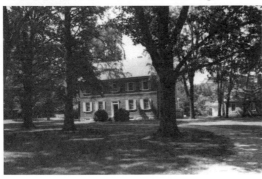

on Blankenbaker in recent years, but it's still ridable. But be careful.

Locust Grove is about halfway through the ride. Club members used to stop and rest there in the gravel driveway in front of the front gate, and have a swig of water and maybe munch on some granola, and contemplate the house.

Locust Grove

It was built in 1790, 10 or so years after Taylor's place, in Georgian style, by George Rogers Clark's brother-in-law. Clark, who founded Louisville and secured the Northwest Territory for the U.S. during the American Revolution, lived here in his old age.

The house is a museum and, with its grounds, is open to public tours.

River Road

Turn left for a nice stretch of River Road, right along the water's edge. You are looking at Indiana on the other shore across about a mile of river.

It's a great place to ride. Unfortunately, automotive traffic has picked up along there in recent years. And it is my opinion that motorists are less friendly there than on practically any other street in Louisville.

That's why I often take the parallel asphalt path that runs through Cox Park to the next turn, which is a left onto Mockingbird Valley Road.

A pedestrian can change direction right into your path with no warning, for example. Also, conflict between cyclists and cars becomes greater at intersections, because neither is necessarily expecting the other. So be careful.

Mockingbird Valley Road

Mockingbird Valley is a great road to ride a bicycle on. It's a moderate climb, to be sure, but it's gently winding and the houses are few, and behind trees and groomed stretches of grass. The world would be a better place if Mockingbird Valley Road were longer.

Frankfort Avenue, Stiltz, and Lexington Road

The stretch that follows is very good practice for Effective Cycling. You're on streets that have a little traffic, but not too much, and some traffic lights to contend with.

Go right on Frankfort and move into the left lane fairly soon. The traffic lights at Hillcrest and Stiltz Avenues are so close together, that it's often less confusing to motor traffic if you get into the left lane before you get to Hillcrest. Then just proceed to the next light and your left turn at Stiltz.

Proceed up Stiltz to Lexington Road, and turn right. Then work your way to the left side of the inside lane to turn left at the light onto Alta Vista.

Shortcut

This ride is designed to take in almost all of Cherokee Park's perimeter roads. But if you don't need that, necessarily, you can save a couple of miles at this point by taking a right at Beals Branch and another right at Scenic Loop, and then bearing left back to Hogan's Fountain.

Louisville's Best

If you don't take the shortcut, though, you will find yourself riding between the beautiful **Louisville Presbyterian Seminary** on the right, and what is, in my opinion, the Louisville area's finest residential neighborhood, on the left.

When you reach Park Boundary Road, you'll see a set of old millstones directly across the street. Those are from an 1817 grist mill operated by a man named Ward, who reportedly was cruel to his slaves. He was not my relative.

Bear right three times, and then left up Golf Course hill. Gear down and just crank on up.

Think of it as a good practice hill—practice for that next hill up to **Hogan's Fountain**, and for life in general. I maintain that if you keep riding around **Cherokee Park**, pretty soon you'll be in good enough shape to ride anywhere.

Route Sheet

0.0	Head east from Hogan's Fountain on Scenic Loop	6.4	Cross Brownsboro
0.4	Straight ahead on Cherokee Road	6.5	Left on Apache Road
		7.0	Springfield - Zachary Taylor Home
0.8	Right on Park Boundary Road	7.1	Right on Blankenbaker Lane
1.0	Bear right	8.3	Locust Grove (Downhill—caution)
1.4	Right after bridge - Seneca Park Road	9.1	Left on River Road
1.7	Bear left up the hill	9.8	Side path option
2.3	Straight on Pee Wee Reese Road	10.8	Left on Mockingbird Valley Road
2.9	Cross Cannons Lane onto Willis Ave.	12.5	Right on Brownsboro Road
		12.9	Left on Reservoir Ave.
3.7	Cross Shelbyville Road onto St. Matthews Ave.	13.4	Right on Frankfort
		13.7	Left on Stilz Ave.
3.8	Jog right, then left, across Westport Road and railroad tracks	14.1	Right on Lexington
		14.6	Left on Alta Vista
		15.6	Right on Park Boundary Road; Bear right next three intersections
4.2	Right on Massie		
4.8	Right on Hubbard's Lane, left on Rudy Lane	17.4	Enter Scenic Loop Bear left all the way back to Hogan's Fountain
5.7	Follow Rudy left	19.0	Finish

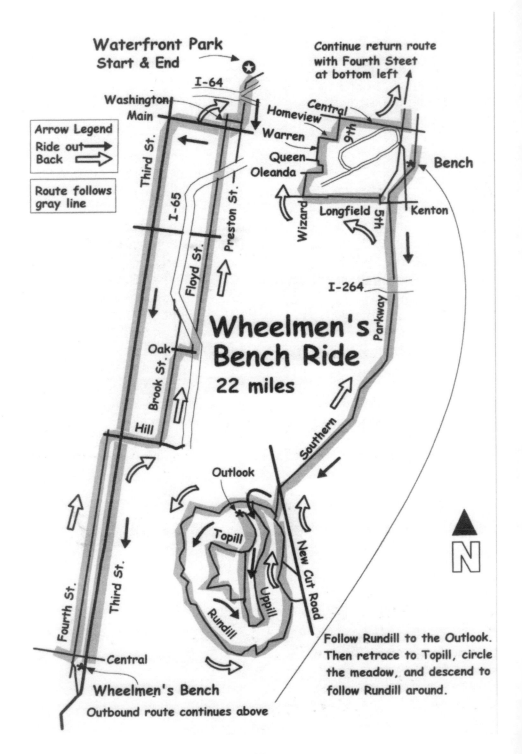

Waterfront Park
Start & End

Continue return route
with Fourth Steet
at bottom left

I-64

Washington
Main

Homeview
Warren
Queen
Oleanda

Central

9th

Bench

Arrow Legend
Ride out
Back

Route follows
gray line

Third St.

I-65

Floyd St.

Preston St.

Wizard

Longfield

5th

Kenton

Oak

Brook St.

I-264

Parkway

Wheelmen's
Bench Ride
22 miles

Hill

Southern

Outlook

New Cut Road

Topill

Uppill

Rundill

Third St.

Fourth St.

N

Central

Wheelmen's Bench

Outbound route continues above

Follow Rundill to the Outlook.
Then retrace to Topill, circle
the meadow, and descend to
follow Rundill around.

Wheelmen's Bench Ride

Twenty-two miles. One significant hill and a few minor ones. Potential for some traffic. Start at Waterfront Park, off River Road near Preston Street.

Cycling had a heyday in Louisville – and, indeed, in the United States and Europe – in the 1890s, that pre-automobile time of bicycles-built-for-two and such. This trip takes in Third Street and Southern Parkway, both popular cycling avenues and fashionable residential streets in those days.

Courier-Journal archives report on two mammoth bicycle parades in the late 1890s – one for the 1896 convention of the League of American Wheelmen, and another the next year to celebrate the opening of a bike path along Southern Parkway.

Both used Third Street, and newspaper accounts reported spectators lining the street several deep from downtown past Eastern Parkway. A lot of the old mansions along Third Street have second or third-floor balconies, and as I ride along there I like to imagine comfortable citizens in period attire relaxing up there to watch the passing wheels.

Staging Area

Start at **Waterfront Park** and proceed up Preston Street to Main Street. Turn right and get on over to the left side of the left lane on Main Street while you have the traffic light to protect your crossing. Turn left at Third Street, and scoot on over to the right side of the right lane there in the same fashion.

Go under the **Convention Center**, being thankful that the City Fathers ultimately decided in the 1990s that it wouldn't be necessary to close Third Street there to enlarge the center.

The stretch of Third from Main to Broadway was the staging area for the big 1897 parade, which ultimately involved 10,000 bicyclists, according to *The Louisville Times*. They were all organized behind marshals in white duck caps and colored sashes.

Many of the cyclists themselves wore colorful garb – club uniforms, clown suits, tramp suits, bloomers. They assembled in the side streets along Third, waiting for the signal to get underway.

Bugles and Cannon Fire

To get that mass moving all at once, parade organizers had arranged for 17 buglers. The head bugler at Broadway was to launch a call, which was to be answered by division buglers back down the street. After the three calls and answers, the whole thing was to roll.

Beyond Broadway, buglers pretty much sounded their horns whenever they felt like it, to help spectators gauge the progress of parade elements.

Meanwhile, on down Third Street in the vicinity of the **Confederate Monument**, the Louisville Board of Park Commissioners waited on a reviewing stand, with a cannon.

They were the parade's honorees. When they heard bugle calls, news accounts said, they would salute with that cannon. *The Times* said bugle calls and cannon fire rang for miles around.

Big Mess

Continue on down Third Street, thankful that you aren't actually in the parade, which sounds fairly disorganized in retrospect, and even tumultuous.

The *Courier-Journal* and *Times* gave it such a buildup in weeks leading up to it, that a lot of people who were scheduled to ride in it, gathered instead on the street south of Broadway to watch it go by.

Captains waiting for their troops back in the staging area delayed the start, and some smart alecks at the front jumped the gun and streaked down the parade route prematurely, to the rambunctious cheers of a crowd that was getting bored.

Some in the crowd assumed the parade was over after those advance elements had passed, and they wandered out onto the street just in time to block the real parade as it got underway.

One marshal clubbed one such obstructionist to the pavement. Small boys ran out from the sidelines and thrust sticks in spokes, bringing cyclists down.

As the parade passed, people from the sidelines jumped on their bikes and joined it, so that – the *Times* reported – the mass included 10,000 cyclists by the time it reached the **Iroquois Cycling Club** clubhouse about where the Watterson Expressway is now.

Monuments

Proceed past the **Confederate Monument** – which was built by church ladies for $12,000 in 1895 and has survived several attempts at removal – and under the railroad underpass just beyond Eastern Parkway.

That underpass is a sort of monument itself, to the dangers of cycling in the old days. It replaced a grade crossing, where, in 1895, Dr. Ed Palmer caught a wheel, fell against a curbstone and was killed.

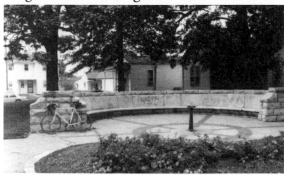

The Wheelmen's Bench

Next comes the **"Wheelmen's Bench,"** a stone seat in **Wayside Park** that was built in 1897. It honors A.D. Ruff, an inventor of cycling equipment from Owingsville, Ky., who died in 1896 and left $1,000 to the Kentucky Division of the League of American Wheelmen.

They spent some of it on a tombstone for Ruff in Owingsville, and some on this bench, where old-time cyclists gathered until World War I for rides into the countryside. The modern Louisville Bicycle Club used to meet at the bench for a Fourth of July ride to Elizabethtown by Dixie Highway and back – which reportedly was a favorite ride of the old timers – but has not in recent years.

The club helped the Metro Parks Department restore the bench in 1987.

Map Matters

This is a long, skinny ride with detail required at both ends and in the middle. To keep it all on one map – and keep the map a size that is handy for a stem clip, I had to split it in half and put the top and bottom halves side by side. I included directions for following from one to the other.

And the trip to the top of Iroquois Hill seemed impossible to explain with arrows. So I included a little text. It will make more sense when you get there.

The Boulevard

After a symbolic rest on the bench, proceed on south out Southern Parkway, which was known as **"The Boulevard"** in the 1890s. It was a popular venue for thousands of cyclists on summer nights, many in fancy knickerbockers and cycling skirts – and many on bicycles built for two.

Land for The Boulevard was purchased by **Charles D. Jacob**, a flamboyant, and rich, Louisville mayor who wanted it for an impressive approach to **Iroquois Park**, for which he also purchased the land.

The purchase of the park land was controversial, because Jacob bought it with his own money and sold it to the city, and the park was sometimes known as "Jacob's Folly" in early days.

Southern Parkway was intended to resemble the Champs-Elysees in Paris, so think about that as you pedal along.

It was fashionable, and crowded, cyclists sharing it with carriages and other conveyances. In an 1897 incident that was in the newspapers for more than a year, Mayme Stout, riding on the front of a steer-from-behind tandem, was struck by the harness shaft of a surrey. She died.

Slight Acclivity

Continue south into the park from the end of the parkway and bear right on Rundill Road. Then hang a left on Uppill Road. I'm not sure whether the aristocratic Jacob was involved in those English-sounding names or not. The parks department says they are just a stylish way of stating the obvious.

You might have to go around a barrier at the entrance to Uppill, because it leads to the top of the knob that is Iroquois Park's signature feature and it's closed to automotive traffic most of the week.

> **Safety Note:** Uppill Road is open to cars from 10 a.m. to 8 p.m. on weekends and Wednesday between May 9 and Oct. 22 – in case you want to plan your trip some other time. I have to say, though, that cars have never been a problem for me, even when they have access.

You are in for a slight acclivity – or "upward slope," as the dictionary defines a word I use here to avoid saying, "You're going to be riding for a mile uphill here."

It is very deceptive, though. It's a gradual slope and a really easy climb if you're not in too high a gear. Your friends will be impressed that you climbed it, and it will be your secret and mine that it is really easy.

Forested Splendor

And boy is that climb ever worth it. When **Frederick Law Olmsted** designed Louisville's three big parks, he intended **Iroquois** to represent forested splendor, while **Shawnee** would be flat playing fields, and **Cherokee** rolling creek bottom.

When you're at the top of Iroquois, where a road named Toppill circles a sort of tree-lined meadow, you will feel like you're in the forest primeval. Often there's a breeze to cool you off from the climb.

Before you circle the top, though, follow Uppill Road around to the right, where it becomes Downill for a stretch. It goes out to an overlook, from which you can see downtown Louisville, and other sights, on a clear day. The parks people sometimes trim the trees there so you can get a good view. And sometimes not.

Safety Note: After you ride around that wonderful, isolated, top of the park, head back down Uppill Road, from whence you came. Resist the temptation to let her rip, though. It's a relatively gentle slope, but you could get cranking if you used no brakes at all, and maybe end up in the bushes.

Mini Route

At the bottom of Uppill, take a left and continue around the park on Rundill, for more forested splendor. You'll be reversing the route of the Kentucky Derby festival's **Mini Marathon**, which circles the park before it heads downtown.

Sometimes it's necessary to go around a barrier on the back side of the hill. You'll know you're almost back to Southern Parkway when you get to the **Iroquois Amphitheater,** which has more than 3,500 seats and has seen its share of big-name performers since it was built in 1938.

Take a right where Rundill meets itself, and head back up the Parkway.

Buy Stuff

A short trip off the Parkway to the right at Woodlawn used to take you to the **Tangerine "Worst Food" Restaurant**, where you could get meat loaf specials, bowls of pinto beans, stewed onions with corn bread and the like.

The sign always said it was the worst food in Kentucky, but that was just a gimmick. Alas, as of the summer of 2003, it's another Louisville legend lost.

Pony Lore

The **Wheelmen's Bench** is just a stone's throw from **Churchill Downs**, and it would be a shame to ride in the area without getting a good look at the storied home of the **Kentucky Derby.**

So watch for Kenton Street on the left as you go up the parkway, and make your way over to Longfield Avenue and ride along the back side of the downs. It's the site of a good deal of excitement and nostalgia and dreaminess on the first Saturday in May each year.

You'll see the barns there, and exercise people, and sometimes a pretty expensive horse or two. Hang a right on Wizard Avenue just past Gate 10, and follow the downs boundary around on Oleanda, Warren, and Queen Avenues, and Homeview Drive and 9th Street, before you get to Central Avenue and the front of the race track.

From 9th Street you'll see the main entrance, and the backside of the twin spires and the grandstand and clubhouse, which is kind of a jumble of windows and vents and pipes and things. It always makes me think of the underside of a space ship in the original Star Wars movie.

Fourth Street-

Hang a left from Central and ride up Fourth Street, past the beer joints and restaurants that cater to the non-high rollers who sustain the track on the days other than Derby. It's a bit less tricky to get under the railroad tracks on Fourth than on Third. When you reach Hill Street, turn right.

Buy Stuff

You might consider a tasty whitefish sandwich at the **Hill Street Fish Fry**, operated by Larry and Mary Jo Linker near Brook Street. It's a small place that once was an ice cream stand, and easy to get into and out of while keeping an eye on bikes.

It's open from 10:30 a.m. to 8 p.m. from Tuesday to Thursday; from 10:30 to 9 Friday and from 11 to 8 Saturday. It's closed Sunday and Monday.

Victor Mature and Medicine

Proceed up Brook Street to Oak, where there's a building that once housed a restaurant owned by a young **Victor Mature**, before he went to Hollywood and became Sampson and various Romans, and before the term "hunk" was coined to describe him.

Turn right there and go over a block to Floyd, and turn left. That's to avoid entanglements with I-65 interchanges that take some of the fun out of riding Brook from Broadway north.

Just at Broadway on Floyd, though, there is some interesting sculpture in the **Wave Garden** on the right—if you're not in a hurry.

Floyd will take you through the heart of Louisville's medical center complex, on which the city has increasingly been leaning lately for one of its claims to fame. As you ride through, somebody might be in one of those buildings getting a new heart, or a new hand.

Cross Main Street and turn right at Washington, then left at Preston, and you're soon back at the start.

Route Sheet

0.0	Right on River Road		14.0	Right out of Park
0.2	Straight on Preston		14.2	Straight on Southern Parkway
0.3	Right on Main		15.3	Woodlawn (possible eatery)
0.8	Left on Third		16.4	Left on Kenton
3.3	Pass Confederate Monument		16.5	Right on Fifth, left on Longfield
4.4	Wheelmen's Bench		17.0	Right on Wizard
5.2	Watterson Expressway		17.1	Right on Oleanda, left on Warren
6.9	Straight into Park		17.2	Left on Queen, right on Warren
7.0	Right onto Rundill Road		17.3	Right on Homeview
7.2	Left on Uppill		17.4	Left on 9th
8.3	Straight on Toppill		17.5	Right on Central
8.7	Bear right to overlook		18.0	Left on Fourth
8.9	Overlook. Backtrack on Downill		19.4	Right on Hill
9.1	Right on Toppill, around the top		19.8	Fish Fry, left on Brook
10.0	Right on Uppill, down the hill		20.2	Right on Oak
11.1	Left on Rundill		20.3	Left on Floyd
11.9	Straight on Rundill		21.0	Cross Broadway
12.5	Go around barrier		21.8	Right on Washington
13.5	Amphitheater		21.9	Left on Preston
			22.2	Back at park

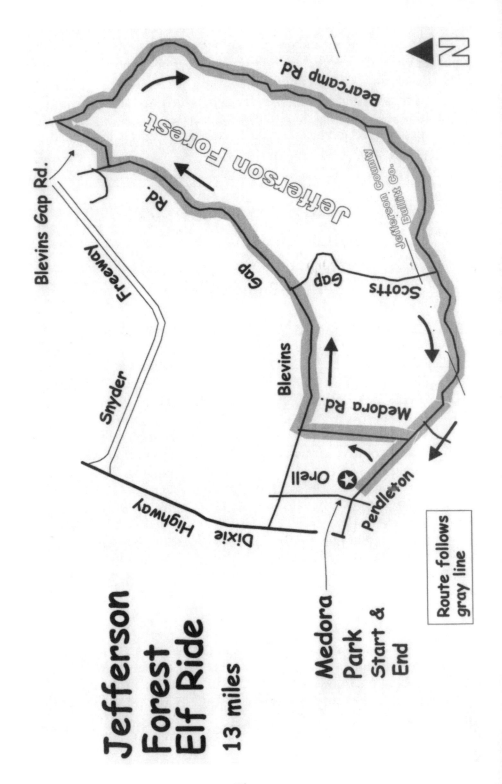

Jefferson Forest Elf Ride

13 miles

Medora Park Start & End

Jefferson Forest

Jefferson County
Bullitt Co.

Blevins Gap Rd.

Freeway

Snyder

Dixie Highway

Orell

Pendleton

Medora Rd.

Blevins Gap Rd.

Scotts Gap

Bearcamp Rd.

Route follows gray line

N

Jefferson Forest Elf Ride

Thirteen miles. One sharp hill and a couple of long gradual ones. Starts at Medora Park, on Pendleton Road, a short distance off Dixie Highway, 2.3 miles south of the Gene Snyder Freeway.

This ride might seem out of sequence because of its length. I judged it more challenging than some of the shorter rides because of one fairly sharp hill, and a couple of long, steady stretches of uphill. They caused my friend Kirk Kandle to grunt a little on his old, 40-pound, bulletproof Schwinn Varsity. But it's very rideable. Good practice hills.

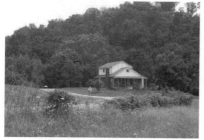

Kirk Kandle on Bearcamp Road

I managed to sneak this ride into a *Courier-Journal* story, along with a couple of others, some years back, when Dwight Stamper was the bike club's touring leader. Dwight was an energetic and innovative officer, with an impish side. Sometimes he was called "Captain America," and he even had a red, white and blue cycling outfit he'd don occasionally.

Dwight had a hand in naming this ride. I can't remember what his exact suggestion was. Suffice it to say there may be elves in the Jefferson Forest. The ride itself is a variation of an old club favorite. It used to start at the Kmart on Outer Loop at New Circle Road, but traffic there makes it less fun now.

It's another ride I enjoy taking people on because they marvel to find something this exquisite off Dixie Highway. It is a true jewel, with stretches of sylvan forest interspersed with some lovely rural homes. It's short enough for fairly new riders, and hilly enough to make them want to get into shape.

Getting There
Start at **Medora Park**, a short distance off Dixie Highway on Pendleton Road. You'll find Pendleton 2.3 miles south of the Snyder Freeway. There's a Dairy Mart on Dixie at its corner with Pendleton, something to make a mental note of in case you want a cold soft drink or a Popsicle after the ride.

The Dairy Mart is at 13401 Dixie, and an A&W Restaurant and Creamery that cyclists have been known to frequent is on down the highway a ways, at 14126.

Hideaways

Head east on Pendleton out of the park, and hang a left on Medora Road. Then turn right on Blevins Gap and start noticing the interesting houses people have tucked away here and there. You might see a volleyball game underway.

There's a steady climb as you head up Blevin's Gap, and just when you get to coast a bit, it suddenly turns right into a good practice hill.

It's easy to miss the turn, in fact. Straight ahead suddenly becomes Stone Street Road, and Blevins Gap makes a right angle turn. If you reach the expressway, you've gone too far.

County Forest

Coast down the other side of the hill, and be ready for a right turn onto Bearcamp Road. Bearcamp sort of bends around and heads back toward Dixie, crossing through chunks of the **Jefferson Forest** and bypassing other chunks.

You'll usually know when you're in the forest. Watch for elves. You're into another steady climb for a ways, but it's never steep, and the downhill is great.

The ride dips into **Bullitt County** on Bearcamp. You'll notice the maintenance boundary, though the road is well kept in both counties.

I call your attention to a couple of trees with incredible roots on the right and left sides of Pendleton Road, which Bearcamp becomes some distance before you reach the railroad tracks as you're getting back toward the park. They are the kind of thing you wouldn't notice if you were whizzing by in a car. A cyclist's bonus.

Stay on Pendleton after the railroad tracks, and you soon find yourself back at **Medora Park.**

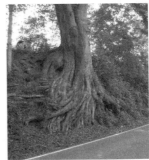

Roots on Pendleton Road

Route Sheet

0.0	East from Medora Park
0.7	Left on Medora Road
1.6	Right on Blevins Gap Road
5.1	Right up the hill on Blevins Gap
5.8	Right on Bearcamp Road
12.7	Pass Medora, bear left on Pendleton
13.4	Back at park

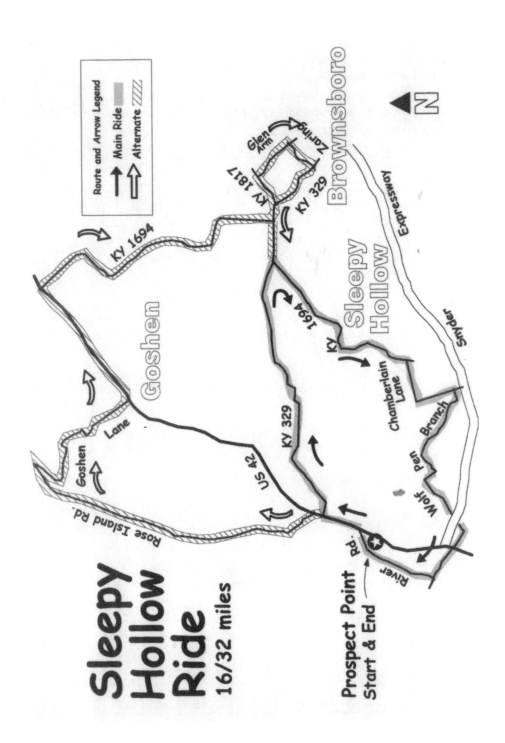

Sleepy Hollow

Sixteen or 32 miles. Two significant hills the short way, and two more the long way. Hilly in general. Potential for traffic in places. Start at Prospect Point Shopping Center parking lot, off U.S. 42, 11 miles northeast of downtown Louisville.

This ride offers two versions of an old club favorite, the second of which was developed to prolong the enjoyment to be had from the first. Both, unfortunately, may be on the endangered list, because of heavy subdivision construction on lovely sections of Chamberlain Lane and Wolf Pen Branch Road, among other places.

The shorter version of this ride has always been sort of a warm up – maybe the first ride in the spring after staying closer to home, or a short ride to enjoy when you don't have time to get out on a real ride.

It's scenic, with a couple of good hills for practice, and some long, gradual ones to build up those slow twitch muscles. Club riders take it in either direction, some preferring one way and others the other.

This ride goes clockwise, which must have been the way somebody first took me.

Downhill Heaven

There's not actually too much to see on either version, except good Kentucky countryside and woods, and some winding roads. Stretches of KY 1694 – one between US 42 and Covered Bridge Road, and the other on Sleepy Hollow Road – are two of my favorite downhill rides anywhere.

Both seem to go on and on. The one on Sleepy Hollow is not as steep as the other, and it winds through shady woods. Both are delightful.

Each crosses a bridge at the bottom, causing my friend David Runge to say, "And you know what that means." It means you have a little climbing practice ahead of you.

Take US 42

You leave the **Prospect Point Shopping Center** parking lot onto River Road, and take a left on US 42 at the light. Traffic can get moving there, but there are four lanes, and it's not usually too menacing. For the short route, hang a right up a short incline onto Covered Bridge Road, also known as KY 329.

It's woodsy and serene almost immediately on Covered Bridge, but you will note that the developers are busy doing something about that. You may get a little traffic on some winding turns in the early going.

Covered Bridge Road climbs sort of gradually to a point near the Oldham County line, and then drops down to **Harrods Creek**, where the actual **covered bridge** – and a **Boy Scout camp** by that name used to be. Both are gone now.

There was a subdivision building boom just inside Oldham County there during the late 1970s when I first started riding that road, and my friend John Bugbee used to ask, "Do you think we should take a poll in this neighborhood on busing?"

Louisville and Jefferson County had just combined and desegregated their schools systems, and the resulting busing for racial balance was controversial.

Waterfalls
The road follows a fork of Harrods Creek as it climbs out of the creek proper, and sometimes in the spring there are very nice waterfalls along there – something to distract you from the conditioning your legs are getting as you pedal up the hill.

Turn right onto KY 1694, also known as Sleepy Hollow Road. The **Sleepy Hollow Golf Course** is on the left a short way down the road. When I rode this route with a group of teenagers that was attached to the Louisville Bicycle Club in the 1980s, they often wanted to stop there for candy and soft drinks.

Any stopping, though, delays the gratification of a great downhill, into the bottom of **Sleepy Hollow**.

Practice Hill
Then you have a pretty good practice hill. Not too steep, but long and winding. It usually is shady. The youth group noted that people we saw carrying jugs of water into the woods along the hill might have illicit crops back in there somewhere.

Turn right on Chamberlain Lane just after the top of the hill, and follow it around past what used to be sod farms and now are subdivisions, and turn right on Wolf Pen Branch Road.

There is some nice leafy coasting and climbing along Wolf Pen Branch, with a pretty good climb from the branch itself. There's an **old mill** off to the right there, in the woods, that was still turning out corn meal after World War II. You can't see it from the road.

Sallie Bingham, author and media heir, bought the mill and the farm that goes with it in the 1980s, and created an easement that will preserve the property.

The road winds around to the left from the top of the hill above the branch, and brings you into subdivision heaven. It climbs a short hill back to US. 42.

Safety Note: Cross the highway for a coast down to River Road, but resist the impulse to spare the brakes. The hill becomes steep as it nears the bottom, and there is a sharp right turn there, with potential for traffic from three directions (counting what might be coming down the road behind you). So be careful.

The right turn on River Road takes you across **Harrods Creek** and back to the start.

Henry's Ark

If you choose the longer version of the ride, you go past the Covered Bridge Road turn off, and turn left on Rose Island Road instead, a short distance farther up U.S. 42.

Ride down the hill around a picturesque small church, and you find yourself viewing an assortment of animals from several continents, including camels and buffalo, various kinds of goats, and exotic birds.

That's **Henry's Ark**, brought to you by **Henry Wallace**, who lives in the farmhouse up the hill. He is a son of Tom Wallace, who was a noted *Courier-Journal* and *Louisville Times* editor through much of the last century up into the 1950s.

Henry Wallace was himself a correspondent for *Time* and *Life* magazines. He lived in Cuba during the 1940s and '50s, and interviewed Ernest Hemingway, among others.

He and his first wife, Netherlands-born Sonja de Vries, were admirers of Fidel Castro. Besides his ark, Henry is known for writing articulate, left-leaning letters to the editor.

Early Family Resort

Rose Island Road used to go to a landing on the Ohio River where regular ferries hauled visitors across to **Rose Island**, actually a peninsula in Clark County on the Indiana side. According to the *Louisville Encyclopedia*, Rose Island had a heyday in the 1920s and 1930s, with a hotel, cottages, a dining hall, swimming pool and dance floor, among other things.

The *Encyclopedia* says the resort advertised a ferry departure every 10 minutes. Rose Island never reopened after the 1937 flood.

Follow Rose Island Road on its winding way through trees and over hills past **Harmony Landing** to a sharp switchback about six and a third miles out, that takes it up a steep hill onto Goshen Lane. It's a fairly significant hill, but winding and shady. Use a low gear.

That takes you back up to US 42 at Goshen.

The **Goshen General Store**, which still has a pot bellied stove, is a pleasant place to stop for a soft drink or a sandwich. Hours are 7 a.m. to 6 p.m. Monday through Friday, and 7 to 3 on Saturday. It's closed on Sunday.

Horse Country

Ride on out US 42 about two and a half miles, and turn right on KY 1694. That is **Hermitage Farm** on the right along there, Louisville's best known thoroughbred farm.

Visitors come to town knowing Louisville is the home of the **Kentucky Derby**, and ask to see the horse farms. Louisvillians have to say most of them are over around Lexington. But Hermitage Farm, operated for years by the late Warner Jones—a long-time chairman of the board at Churchill Downs—is close enough.

In 1985, Jones sold one horse, a colt called Seattle Dancer, by Nijinski II, for $13.1 million.

The route goes down the back side of Hermitage Farm, and commences a lovely coast into the valley of Harrods Creek. The climb out is long, but it is gradual and not too steep.

Spice Cake

Turn left on KY 369, and then bear left onto KY 1817 where the two meet about three tenths of a mile farther on. It's kind of a tricky fork, with traffic on 369 coming around a curve into the intersection, so use caution.

Take 1817 to Glenarm Road and take a right turn, then turn right again on Zaring Road. That will bring you out to KY 329 and the village of

Brownsboro. The **Brownsboro General Store** has added "and Eaterie," to its name, and now keeps peculiar hours for a general store. It does a split shift for lunch and dinner now and is closed Sundays. Lunch hours are 11 a.m. to 2 p.m. Monday through Saturday. Dinner hours are 5:30 to 7:30 p.m. Tuesday through Thursday, and they stretch to 8 p.m. on Friday and Saturday. No dinner on Monday.

But you can still get that wonderful apple spice cake that they've sold for years.

Take KY 369 back to KY 1694. Pass on by the stretch of 1694 you came out on—which will be on your right—and ride down to a stretch of the same road that takes off on the left a short distance farther. Turn left and follow the same route as the short version of this ride back to **Prospect Point**.

Route Sheet

0.0	Leave Prospect Point shopping center
0.1	Left on US 42
0.8	Right on Covered Bridge Road
5.7	Right on Sleepy Hollow Road (KY 1694)
7.9	Big Hill
9.1	Right on Chamberlain Lane
10.5	Right on Wolf Pen Branch Road
14.1	Cross US 42 onto River Creek Road
14.7	Right on River Road at the bottom of the hill
16.4	Back at start

Alternative Route

0.0	Leave Prospect Point shopping center
0.1	Left on US 42
0.9	Left on Rose Island Road
6.3	Right on Goshen Lane, up the big hill
9.0	Left on US 42
11.5	Right on KY 1694
16.5	Left on KY 369
16.8	Left on KY 1817
17.5	Right on Glenarm Road
18.3	Right on Zaring Road
18.9	Right on KY 329 at Brownsboro
19.9	Straight on KY 329
20.8	Left on 1694
23.0	Big hill
24.2	Right on Chamberlain Lane
25.6	Right on Wolf Pen Branch
29.2	Cross US 42 onto River Creek Road
29.7	Right on River Road at the bottom of the hill
31.6	Back at start

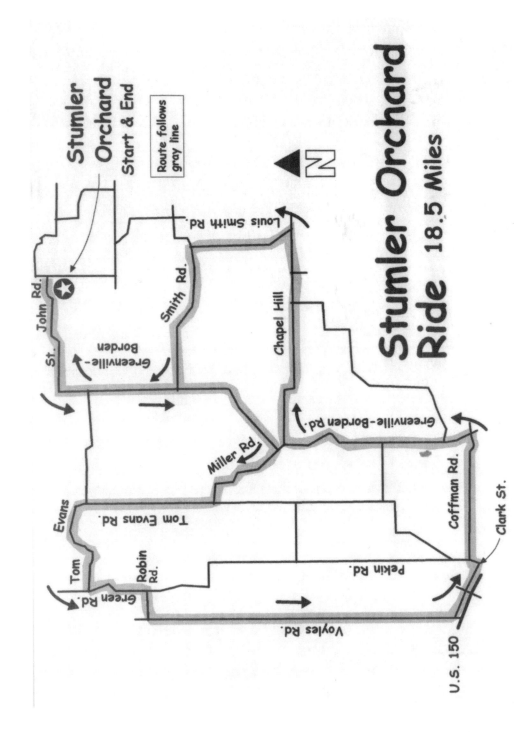

Stumler Orchard
Start & End

Route follows gray line

Stumler Orchard
Ride 18.5 Miles

N

Louis Smith Rd.

Smith Rd.

Chapel Hill

John Rd.

St.

Greenville-Borden

Greenville-Borden Rd.

Coffman Rd.

Clark St.

Miller Rd.

Evans

Tom Evans Rd.

Tom

Pekin Rd.

Robin Rd.

Green Rd.

Voyles Rd.

U.S. 150

Stumler Orchard Ride

> Nineteen Miles. Mild hills. Potential for traffic, especially in fall and spring. Begin at Stumler Orchard, on St. Johns Road in Clark County, Ind., about 20 miles from downtown Louisville. Take I-64 from Louisville to the US 150-Greenville-Paoli exit. Take 150 to Navilleton Road, and follow the Huber and Stumler orchard signs.

Stumler is one of two well-known orchards on the bench above the knob hills in Indiana, across the Ohio River from Louisville. The other, **Huber Orchard and Winery**, is the starting point for another ride later in the book.

Both are very pleasant rides in rural Indiana. Both orchards are direct-to-the consumer farm operations that draw a lot of customers from the Louisville area.

The Stumler farm is very busy in the fall, especially on the first full weekend in October when 20,000 people show up for the annual **Applefest**. There can be a bit of weekend traffic at strawberry time from mid-May to mid-June, too.

You probably will enjoy this ride more at other times of year, on weekdays, or at least early in the day if you're riding at peak times. You can cut off the highest-traffic portion of this ride by taking the Miller Road Cutoff, described below, and sacrificing a couple of miles of the route.

Veggie City

Stumler Orchard is a great place to stock up on fresh vegetables from May to December. The farm market is open from 9 a.m. to 6 p.m.

There also is a family restaurant that is open year round, though on Friday, Saturday and Sunday only, from January through March. Hours then are 11 a.m. to 9 p.m. Friday and Saturday, and 9 a.m. to 6 p.m. Sunday. For the rest of the year, they add 11 a.m. to 8 p.m. hours daily. You can get a bowl of beans with cornbread there that is the perfect lunch after a nice morning ride.

Stumler also has a petting zoo, tours to the pumpkin patch and such. It's a very festive place in the fall.

Rural Splendor

This is just a nice, fairly easy ride out through lush Hoosier farm country. There are just enough hills to keep it interesting, and just enough dogs to give you somebody to talk to.

Head west on St. John Road, meander past an interesting country cemetery. Stop and read a few stones if you have time. Turn left on the Greenville-Borden Road.

You make a right turn on Miller Road, follow that over to Tom Evans Road, and make another right. Tom Evans passes Temple Road and then turns to the left. A couple of miles later it tees into Green Road, and you turn left again.

About a half-mile down Green Road, Robin Road takes off on the right and crosses over a couple of tenths of a mile to Voyles Road. Take that and follow Voyles all of the way into Greenville.

Turn left on Clark Street to avoid U.S. 150, which can be pretty busy. If you're thirsty for a soft drink or hungry, though, you can follow Cross Street a short distance to the right, cross 150, and make a stop at the **Greenville Mini-Mart.**

Buy Stuff

The Mini-Mart opens at 4 a.m. every day but Sunday, in case you're an early riser, and stays open until 10 p.m. On Sunday they don't open until 6 a.m.

When you're back on Clark Street, take a left at Pekin Road, and a right almost immediately on Arthur Coffman Road.

Safety Note: Coffman is a delightful road, but it takes a kind of sharp and twisty downhill after about a mile, and you're barely at the bottom of the hill when you want to turn left onto Greenville-Borden Road. So be careful.

Short Cut

If you look at the ride map at all, you will notice that the right turn you take on Chapel Hill Road is not very far from where you turned off Greenville-Borden, onto Miller, earlier in the ride.

If you want to make this a 16-mile ride instead of an 19-mile one, here's your chance. And if, on the drive up to Stumler, you noticed a lot of traffic on Chapel Hill and Louis Smith Roads, such a short cut might not be a bad idea. Just continue straight on, and backtrack on St. John to Stumler.

Chapel Hill, Louis Smith and Smith Roads are nice in ordinary times, though, and that extra couple of miles will help burn off that bean soup and corn bread you've maybe been thinking about the whole ride.

If you choose that option, go right on Chapel Hill, left on Louis Smith Road, and left again on Smith Road. A short distance down Smith road you'll see a picturesque old Hoosier farm house on a hill to the right, and it says "Louis Smith" on the mail box.

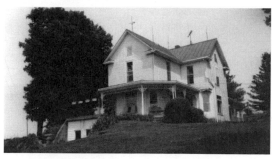

Louis Smith house

I guess it could be *the* Louis Smith. Climb and wind a bit, and then turn right on Greenville-Borden, and right again on St. John, and you're back at Stumler.

Route Sheet

0.0	Leave Stumler on St. John Rd.
1.0	Left on Greenville-Borden Rd.
3.1	Right on Miller Rd.
3.9	Right on Tom Evans Rd, Follow it around to left
5.9	Left on Green Rd.
6.4	Right on Robin Rd.
6.6	Left on Voyles Rd.
9.2	Left on Clark St.
9.4	Cross Cross St., Store to right
9.7	Left on Pekin Rd., Right on Coffman Rd.
10.8	Left on Greenville-Borden Rd.
12.5	Right on Chapel Hill
14.4	Left on Louis Smith
15.2	Left on Smith
16.5	Right on Greenville-Borden
17.5	Right on St. John
18.6	Finish at Stumler

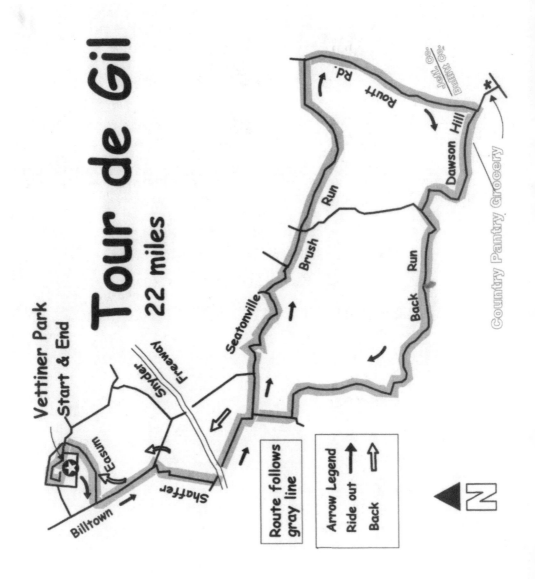

Tour de Gil
22 miles

Vettiner Park
Start & End

Billtown

Easum

Shaffer

Snyder Freeway

Seatonville

Brush Run

Back Run

Routt Rd.

Dawson Hill

Josh Gap

Bullitt Gap

Country Pantry Grocery

Route follows gray line

Arrow Legend
Ride out
Back

N

Tour de Gil

Twenty-two miles. One significant hill, and some rollers. Start at Charlie Vettiner Park, off Billtown Road two miles south of Jeffersontown, or about the same distance north of the Gene Snyder Freeway.

This ride is a Louisville Bicycle Club favorite, named after **Gil Morris**, proprietor of **Louisville's Highland Cycle, Inc.**, and a sort of patron saint of the club.

This is Gil's ride, one he used to do every morning before work, to keep reminding himself during some lean years why he was in the bicycle business.

He didn't name it, though. The name was applied by one of the riders he invited to ride along, riders who became a group that eventually reached the hundreds on Wednesday evenings several times a year.

Gil would offer drinks, cooled in ice in a canoe, and hot dogs to be roasted on coat hangers at his house in the Fern Creek area, to all comers. He sent out photo copies of hand-lettered invitations that are famous for their illegibility, and for their prejudice against "red stuff"—or ketchup —which he would not offer for the hotdogs.

The ride became a club staple, attended by old-timers and new riders alike, and has even been considered neutral ground for feuding factions in the club.

Under New Management

Gil, 75 now, has some dizziness from head injuries received when a robber beat him in his store a few years back. So he hasn't been able to ride the route himself in recent years. And in 2002, ill health forced him to give up sponsoring it entirely.

The club has kept it on the ride schedule, though, moving it to **Vettiner Park**, which is not far from Gil's place, and riding forth in Gil's honor.

Our Link to the Past

The **Louisville Bicycle Club** claims a founding date of 1897. But Gil says that is a "romanticization" of the facts. Actually, he and some customers started the modern club in 1957 or so. But he is himself a sort of club link to the 1890s heyday of cycling in Louisville and elsewhere, through his connection with Howard Jefferis.

Jefferis had a shop on "Bicycle Row" in downtown Louisville in the 1890s, and his brother, Tom, was a racing cyclist who enjoyed celebrity along lines of that now enjoyed by baseball players.

The heyday faded fast after the turn of that century, and Jefferis moved his shop out to Bardstown Road in 1911, and then held on in the business into his old age.

One day in 1940 when Gil was 13, he rode his two-speed Schwinn Paramount past Jefferis' shop, and Jefferis yelled after him, "Hey, kid. You want a job?"

Passing on the Legacy

Gil said Jefferis tried to make a racer of him, and failed. But he showed Gil many of the routes the old timers rode, and which the club now rides. And variations of which show up quite a bit in this book. Jefferis said a small contingent of riders from the heyday was still doing rides around Louisville up until World War I.

The old cyclist died when Gil was 17, and Gil took over the shop, which is still in the same building, though it has taken over some nearby

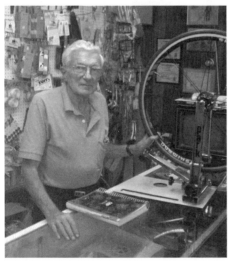

Gil Morris

space, too. Gil kept riding through years when most people no longer did, and kept selling bicycles through a lot of lean times, punctuated by the occasional boom.

He and a couple of customers started going on fairly regular weekend rides again in the 1950s, and eventually posted a list of rides and times in his bike shop, so that others could join them. They put the name "Louisville Wheelmen" at the top of the list. That was the local club's name until it was changed in 1996.

The club has grown to a membership of more than 500 as this book was being written, and it schedules rides all year around, virtually every day in the summer.

Bending to Progress

The Tour de Gil originally went out Billtown Road from Gil's house on Waltlee Road, onto Shaffer Lane and down Seatonville Road, left on Routt Road and back to Waltlee via Taylorsville Road and Billtown Road.

A bridge went out on Routt Road, though, where it crosses the Floyds Fork of the Salt River near Taylorsville Road, and wasn't immediately replaced. Gil said traffic was getting kind of heavy on Taylorsville Road anyway. So he took the tour in a less busy direction, and this ride follows it.

Head out the back side of Vettiner Park onto Easum Road, and follow it around to Billtown Road. The traditional Tour de Gil has taken Billtown straight out to Seatonville Road for years, but this version will take a right on Shaffer Lane, to get out of traffic.

Go left at Seatonville Road, and left again where KY 1115 comes in, and then down the big Seatonville Hill. It's long and winding. Be careful.

Countryside

From the bottom of the hill, Seatonville goes on through rural Jefferson County, past farms and streams and old graveyards, and you quickly see why this became a favorite ride.

At Echo Trail, the name of the road changes to Brush Run Road, and the route follows it on to a landmark rural fire station at its corner with Routt Road. Turn right and proceed through a series of roller hills, to Dawson Hill Road.

Turn right on Dawson hill. The road itself turns right a couple of miles later, but you stay straight on Back Run Road, which is also designated KY 1115.

Smallville

The Tour de Gill lost a major element of charm a few years back when the old bridge that took Back Run across the Floyds Fork was replaced. The new bridge came with a new piece of road that bypassed a collection of vacation-type homes that had been clustered around the old bridge.

The buildings were small and had some fancy trim, which caused somebody in the club—Gil thinks it was one-time president Jay Abraham— to call the place the **Gingerbread Village**.

But my friend Dominic Bosco told me that friends of his in high school believed the place was called **Smallville**, and that little people would come out of the houses when no one was looking.

He said a friend of his even sneaked up on Smallville once, hoping to steal a tiny t-shirt off a clothesline to prove the existence of the little people.

Gingerbread Hill

Anyway, anybody who is on a second or later Tour de Gil—or any of the many other rides that use that route—knows crossing the **Floyds Fork** means it's time to get ready for a pretty good practice hill that takes Back Run back up to Seatonville Road.

The first time I ever climbed that hill I happened to be riding beside Jean Nave, a noted Louisville cyclist who had led international cycling trips in Kentucky.

Jean said the way to climb a hill is to ignore it. Just look at your front wheel, she said, and begin repeating, "One little two little three little Indians." Work all of the way up to ten, and then start back, "Ten little nine little eight little Indians." And then go back up and so forth, and pretty soon you're at the top of the hill.

Worked for me.

Wrap it Up

You bear left onto Seatonville at the end of Back Run Road, and then take a right on Shaffer Lane. Take a left on Billtown Road, and a right on Easum Road, and then turn left back into the park.

The ride used to end at Gil's place, and then we'd eat and drink and sometimes catch up with bike riders we didn't see on any other rides. That might continue elsewhere with the club-sponsored Tours de Gil. But it won't be the same.

Route Sheet

0.0	Head for the back side of Charlie Vettiner Park
0.7	Right on Easum Road
1.6	Left on Billtown Road
2.4	Right on Shaffer Lane
3.2	Left on Seatonville Road
4.1	Left on Seatonville Road
4.8	Big, twisty, downhill
6.3	Pass Echo Trail, Seatonville becomes Brush Run Road
9.1	Right on Routt Road (KY 1531)
11.3	Right on Dawson Hill Road
13.0	Dawson Hill becomes Back Run Road
16.2	Gingerbread Hill
17.4	Left on Seatonville Road
18.5	Right on Shaffer Lane
19.3	Left on Billtown Road
20.1	Right on Easum Road
21.0	Left into park
21.7	Back at start

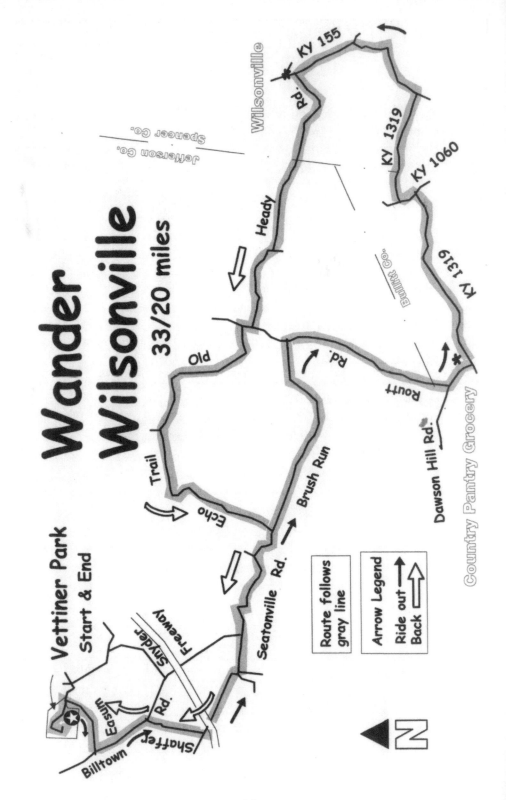

Wander Wilsonville
33/20 miles

Vettiner Park
Start & End

Wilsonville

Jefferson Co.
Spencer Co.

Bullitt Co.

KY 155
KY 1319
KY 1060
KY 1319

Wilsonville Rd.

Heady

Old

Trail

Echo

Brush Run

Routt Rd.

Dawson Hill Rd.

Country Pantry Grocery

Seatonville Rd.

Snyder Freeway

Easum Rd.

Shaffer

Billtown

Route follows gray line

Arrow Legend
Ride out
Back

N

Wander Wilsonville

Thirty-three miles with a 20-mile alternative. One significant hill, and some rollers. Start at Charlie Vettiner Park, off Billtown Road two miles south of Jeffersontown, or about the same distance north of the Gene Snyder Freeway.

This ride itself is offered as a sort of alternative to the traditional Tour de Gil, which follows roads where a lot of building is going on, and which, alas, may not be too much fun to ride much longer.

It takes some of the less-traveled Tour de Gil roads and adds some that have the same flavor, but are a little farther out. It includes a proposed "alternative to the alternative" that skips all but the least traveled Tour de Gil Roads.

That ride would start and end at **Country Pantry Grocery** at the corner of Dawson Hill Road and KY 1319. You can usually park there, but it is necessary to check with someone at the store first, to find out where your vehicle will be out of the way.

Tour de Gil Plus

This ride starts out on the same route as the Tour de Gil, which precedes it in this book. Get on Easum Road at the backside of **Vettiner Park**, and then take Billtown and Shaffer to Seatonville Road, continue on Brush Run Road and turn right on Routt Road.

Be careful on that long, twisty downhill on Seatonville Road. At least one club member has been overtaken by glee there, only to find herself catapulted over the guard rail where the road turns left at the bottom.

When Routt Road reaches Dawson Hill Road, turn left to KY 1319. **The Country Pantry** is on that corner. Its hours are from 5 a.m. to 9 p.m. Monday through Friday, from 7 to 9 on Saturday, and from 8 to 7 on Sunday.

Turn left on KY 1319 and take that wonderful long downhill to **Plum Creek**. Turn left again just across the creek. The road remains KY 1319, though KY 1060 takes off to the right there.

KY 1319 winds around a bit and then reaches KY 155, where you turn left.

Volleyball, Anyone?

KY 155 takes you into **Wilsonville**, where you watch for a left turn onto Old Heady Road.

There isn't much to Wilsonville that is visible to the eye, but my friend David Runge insists there is an underground volleyball factory around there somewhere. He says Wilson, the volleyball that was such a friend to Tom Hanks in the movie *Cast Away*, was made there.

He says he can hardly ever get anybody to believe him, though.

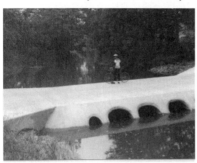

Bridge over Plum Creek

There's an interesting concrete bridge across Plum Creek about half a mile along on Old Heady that requires caution during high water times. Turn right across it and continue on a delightful road.

You jog right for a ways when you come to Routt Road, but turn left then and continue on Old Heady. Its name will change to Echo Trail when you pass Thurman Road.

Almost four miles later, you reach Seatonville Road, where you turn right and retrace your steps up the Seatonville hill, and back by Shaffer and Billtown to the park.

As you climb that long, twisty hill, just remember how much fun it was to come down.

If you're on the alternative ride, you turn left on Seatonville, right on Routt Road, and left on Dawson Hill back to the store.

Route Sheet

0.0	Head for the back side of Charlie Vettiner Park
0.7	Right on Easum Road
1.6	Left on Billtown Road
2.4	Right on Shaffer Lane
3.2	Left on Seatonville Road
4.1	Left on Seatonville Road
4.8	Big, twisty, downhill
6.3	Pass Echo Trail, Seatonville becomes Brush Run Road
9.1	Right on Routt Road (KY 1531)
11.3	Left on Dawson Hill Road
11.8	Country Pantry, left on KY 1319
14.3	Left on KY 1319
17.1	Left on KY 155
18.0	Wilsonville, left on Old Heady Road
18.5	Right across concrete bridge
21.6	Right on Routt Road
21.7	Left on Old Heady Road
22.3	Pass Thurman Road, Old Heady becomes Echo Trail
26.1	Right on Seatonville
27.6	Seatonville Hill
28.3	Right on Seatonville
29.4	Right on Shaffer Lane
30.2	Left on Billtown Road
31.0	Right on Easum Road
31.9	Left into park
32.6	End

Buffalo Run
25 miles

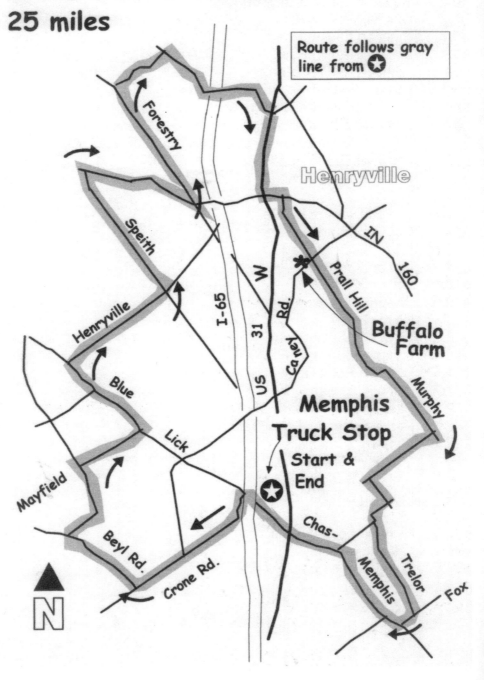

Route follows gray line from ⭐

Henryville

Forestry

Speith

IN 160

Prall Hill

Buffalo Farm

Henryville

Blue

I-65

W

31

US

Caney Rd.

Murphy

Memphis Truck Stop
Start & End

Lick

Mayfield

Beyl Rd.

Crone Rd.

Chas-Memphis

Trelor

Fox

N

Buffalo Run

Twenty-four miles. Very few hills. Start at the Country Style Plaza truck stop, on the right side of I-65, about 16 miles north of Louisville.

I love riding in the southern Indiana counties across the Ohio River from Louisville, and have done a lot of it over the years. But about every ride I try seems to encounter a significant hill somewhere.

I run into hills like **Tunnel Mill** or those coming out of **Bethlehem**, or **Finley Knob** and such. My friend Marilyn Motsch, a Louisville graphic artist and noted cyclist, on the other hand, seems good at finding rides without any really big hills.

All rides have hills, of course—except Turtle Rides, and even those have the occasional acclivity. Hills are a part of cycling. They make you stronger.

My friend David Runge refers to hills as "altitude adjustment opportunities." You build those hill-climbing legs on hills, and the legs give you freedom to ride wherever you want.

But it is fun once in awhile to go out on a ride where you don't have to worry about a quick shift into that really low gear and a long stretch of grinding.

So I've chosen two of Marilyn's rides for the book—this one and the Lanesville Ride a little later on. I'm not saying they don't have hills, just that you shouldn't ever have to look up and think, "Oh no."

Buffalo Man

The buffalo on this ride, all seven of them, belong to **Donnie Guthrie**, of **Henryville**. Guthrie kind of snorted when I asked about his "buffalo farm." Apparently he doesn't think of it as such.

According to **Butch Furnish**—owner of **Furnish's Marathon & Wrecker Service** in Henryville and the man who referred me to Guthrie— Guthrie is a sort of bargain-hunter, a man who buys and swaps and trades things.

Guthrie said he got the buffalo on a sealed bid from the state, because they were a good deal. He had priced buffalo and he entered a bid that was a bargain, and he got them.

99

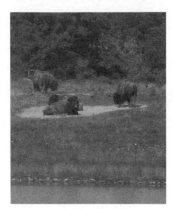

Don Guthrie's buffalo

But then he had the buffalo. "They've kind of messed my place up," he said. But he said when this book was being written that he'd had them for three years, and planned to keep them awhile longer.

So you should see them on the right when you get to the corner of Prall Hill Road and Caney Road.

Country Style Plaza

But the buffalo don't come until near the end of the ride, at about mile 16. Start at the **Country Style Plaza truck stop**. It's one of the outlying places where the bike clubs have started rides in recent years to get beyond traffic.

Marilyn actually has started her ride a bit south, at **Silver Creek High School**, but I moved it for this book to eliminate a stretch of US 31.

Take a right out of the truck stop and cross under the Interstate, and turn left on Crone Road. Follow that down a couple of miles to Beyl Road, turn right and follow it around a turn over to Mayfield Road.

Wander Indiana

Indiana roads seem to change names without notice, and sometimes go back and forth between names. Some maps call a chunk of Beyl Road— where you turn right about 1 mile after you first turn onto Beyl Road— William Boiling Road. It's hard to miss it, in any case.

It is nice riding along here, through farms and new residential building. A right on Mayfield takes you over to Blue Lick Road, where you turn left and go over to Henryville Road. Turn right, and then left on Speith Road, and back right on IN 160.

Just before the overpass that would take you back over I-65, hang a left onto Forestry Road. It takes you into a chunk of **Clark County State Forest.**

Portage in the Trees

About a mile and a half up Forestry Road, you'll see a stretch of gravel on your right that leads to a barricade intended to keep automotive traffic from entering the state forest at this point.

But that doesn't mean you. You're on a bicycle. Unless it's a mountain bike, with fat tires, you might want to dismount and push it the 60 or 70 yards past the barricade and onto a paved forest road. Actually, you might want to even if it is a mountain bike.

Take that road to the right, and enjoy the trees. The Clark forest is Indiana's oldest state forest, established in 1903 on part of land once given to **George Rogers Clark** for his service in the Revolutionary War. Experimental planting began here in 1904, and the forest is considered a national model in scientific forestry.

Henryville

The forest road joins US 31 at the forest entrance, and a right turn takes you a mile or so down to **Henryville**, a town that has long drawn its living from the railroad and highways that go through here.

Furnish, the wrecker man, said it was named for **Henry Ferguson**, called Col. Ferguson in an old history at the Filson Historical Society library in Louisville. Furnish said Ferguson owned a lot of land around town.

You turn left on IN 160 in Henryville, and then right onto Pennsylvania Street, just beyond the railroad tracks. There's a great-looking old mansion on the right across the tracks from the street, with a well-kept yard but in obvious need of repairs on shutters and some other trim.

Centurian Thelma Masters

Thelma Masters, a 100-year-old woman Furnish referred me to as an authority on town history, said the old house was built by a Doctor Ferguson, of the landed family, who had died before she came to town in 1910.

It belongs now to Robert Applegate, whose parents lived there, and who I saw meticulously grooming the grounds one day when I rode past.

Mrs. Masters was a teacher for many years at schools in Henryville and nearby communities and she has a good memory.

She and her friends used to take the train from Henryville to Scottsburg, 10 miles up the line, and go to a movie. The movie would let out in time to catch an Inter-Urban train back home.

She also rode the Inter-Urban across the Big Four Bridge into Louisville for years, going to summer school at the University of Louisville.

The Feed Store

Beyond the old Ferguson house along the tracks is an **old feed mill** that Furnish said flourished because of the railroad, and once was one of the main businesses in town. The business hauled feed for miles around, and brought in coal and distributed it, among other things, he said.

Mrs. Masters said Henryville is far bigger in terms of houses than it was when she came to town, but doesn't have nearly as many businesses.

There used to be a sawmill and a bakery, she said, and a tomato canning factory, whose employees, incidentally, once included Margaret Ann Sanders, mother of Col. Harland Sanders, of Kentucky Fried Chicken fame.

Buy Stuff

And speaking of feed, Henryville is a place where a lot of riders stop to pick up a piece of pie, or even an omlette, at **Schuler's Family Restaurant,** on 160 out by I-65. Hours of operation at Schuler's are 6 a.m. to 9 p.m., seven days a week.

Other places to buy soft drinks, sandwiches and the like include **Tanner's**, on US 31—open from 8 a.m. to 8:30 p.m. Monday through Saturday, and 8 to 6 on Sunday—and **Adams IGA** on Pennsylvania Street. It's open 7 a.m. to 8 p.m. Monday through Saturday, and 8 to 5 on Sunday.

Buffalo

Follow Pennsylvania around to the left. It becomes Prall Hill Road and takes you out past **Donnie Guthrie's place**, where you might see the buffalo on the right, in a field with a pond just before Caney Road.

Guthrie also has an **omnibus** sitting out in the yard, a stage coach version of the modern bus, such as those the giant Jim Porter used to drive in Shippingport and Portland on the other side of the Ohio River.

On past the buffalo and on down the road, take a left on Trelor Road, and then a right on Fox Road, by the log house, and another right on Charlestown-Memphis Road. That will take you through Memphis and back to the truck stop.

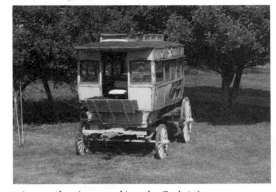

An omnibus (stagecoach) at the Guthries'

Route Sheet

0.0   Leave Country Style Plaza truck stop, right on Blue Lick

0.3   Left on Crone Road

2.2   Right on Beyl Road

3.2   Right on William Boiling (or Beyl) Road

4.3   Right on Mayfield Road

5.1   Left on Blue Lick Road

6.3   Right on Henryville Road

7.7   Left on Speith Road

9.4   Right on IN 160

10.6   Left on Forestry Road

12.2   Walk the bike right around the barricade about 70 yards, onto forest road, and turn right

12.9   Bear left

13.1   Bear right

14.5   Out park entrance and right on US 31W

15.2   Left on IN 160 in Henryville

15.5   Right on Pennsylvania Street, after the railroad tracks. It turns left and becomes Prall Hill, then Murphy Road, and turns a couple of more times

16.5   Buffalo on right, near Caney Road

20.6   Left on Trelor Road

21.8   Right on Fox Road, by log house

22.0   Right on Charlestown-Memphis Road

24.3   Back at truck stop

Mitchell Hill Ride
26 miles

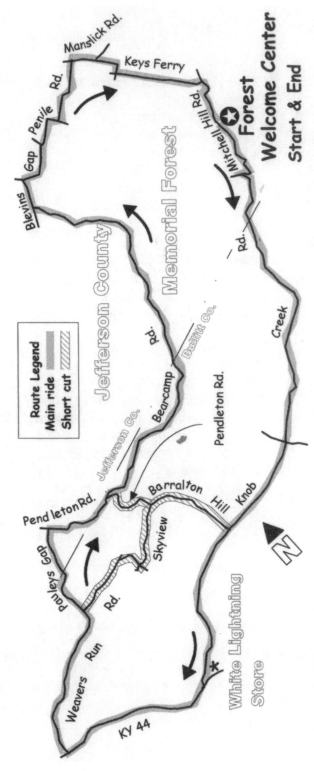

Route Legend
Main ride
Short cut

Forest Welcome Center
Start & End

Memorial Forest

Jefferson County

Bullitt Co.

Jefferson Co.

Manslick Rd.

Keys Ferry

Penile Gap Rd.

Blevins

Mitchell Hill Rd.

Rd.

Creek

Pendleton Rd.

Bearcamp

Rd.

Pendleton Rd.

Barralton

Skyview

Hill

Knob

Danleys Gap

Run

Rd.

Weavers

KY 44

White Lightning Store

N

104

Mitchell Hill Ride

Twenty-six miles, more or less. At least one significant hill; more if you choose. Start at the Jefferson County Memorial Forest Welcome Center, on Mitchell Hill Road. Take the Gene Snyder Freeway to the Fairdale Exit, drive into Fairdale, turn right on New Cut Road, and left immediately on Mitchell Hill Road. The Welcome Center is about a mile and three quarters out, across from the entrance to Tom Wallace Park.

Most beginning riders don't like hills much, because it's hard to climb hills at first, and one has to wrestle with self doubt about whether you'll actually make it up the hill, and it's just different from the freedom of riding along without much effort.

But hill climbing is like a lot of other endeavors, more fun when you have developed the skill to do it—sometimes especially when you can see that you can do it better than other people.

It's a matter of learning and conditioning, knowing what gear to be in and when to shift, and building some leg muscle. And there really is only one way to achieve both. Go out and climb some hills.

That's what this ride is for. I was going to call it the Practice Hill ride, but I was afraid you'd be onto me on that one by now, and would just skip past it. You shouldn't. This ride is good for you. If, every time you started thinking that hill climbing is a tough thing to do, you would go and do this ride, pretty soon it wouldn't be so tough anymore.

Up, Up and Away

In the spirit of grabbing the bull by the horns, the first thing this ride does is climb up Mitchell Hill. Leave the Welcome Center parking lot, turn left and get ready to climb.

Mitchell Hill is a pretty good hill, but it's not the worst hill in the world. Some club members measure hills by the notorious **Pottershop Hill** on the century version of the **Old Kentucky Home Tour**—a September Louisville Bicycling Club invitational.

Some see the toughness of Pottershop as merely a challenge—a challenge to go out and find tougher hills, and inflict them on others. There's a rumored monster hill that comes out of Westport, Kentucky to US 42.

There's a climb up Buck Creek Road in Trimble County that adds what my friend David Runge calls "texture" to a long, steep climb.

Easy Stuff

But I'm not trying to inflict anything on you here. I just want you to climb this one big hill, for practice, and then complete the rest of the 26 miles of the ride pretty much unmolested by hills.

You take Knob Hill Road down the other side of Mitchell Hill and follow it on down to KY 44. You can double back a tenth of a mile on 44 if you like, and stop at **Goldsmith's White Lightning** store for soft drinks and sandwiches.

Hours at the White Lightning are 6 a.m. to 10 p.m. Monday through Thursday, 6 to 11 Friday and Saturday, and 7 to 10 on Sunday.

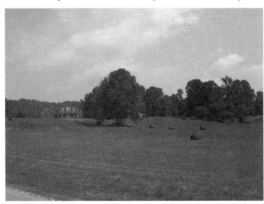
Country scene on Pendleton Road

Continue on 44 to Weavers Run Road and turn right. Weavers Run turns right again after a couple of miles, but you stay straight on Pauleys Gap Road. Then turn right on Pendleton Road. That also turns right in a bit, but you stay straight on Bear Camp Road.

Follow that to Blevins Gap Road, and turn right there and on Penile and Manslick Roads. Manslick bears to the left after awhile, but you stay straight on Keys Ferry Road, which takes you back to Mitchell Hill Road— where a right turn takes you back to the start.

Piece o' cake.

Unless You *Want* Exercise

If, on the other hand, you're serious about wanting to build your hill-climbing skills, this ride does offer opportunity along those lines in a selection of short cuts.

At about six and a half miles into the ride, for example, you could take a right onto Barralton Hill Road and climb about a mile to a knob the map calls **Pendleton Hill**. You could drop down the other side on Pendleton Road and hit Bearcamp

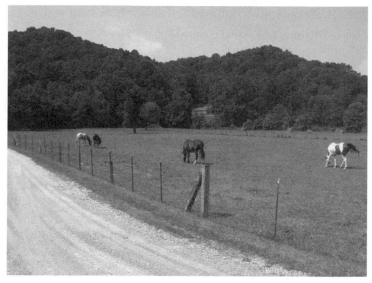

Hills on Pendleton Road

Road and be back to the start in 20 miles.

Next to Pendleton Hill is another prominence the maps call **Cundiff Hill**. You get to it by staying on the original route to KY 44 and following Weavers Run to the right where it leaves Pauleys Gap Road. Once at the top, you could take a left on Skyview Drive—which offers a nice vista, incidentally—and drop down to Bearcamp with a left on Pendleton, and get back to the start in, uh, 28 miles.

A Number of Possible Combinations

OK, that would be in the way of a negative shortcut. But we're talking hill climbing opportunities here. You could do the same thing, only turn right off Skyview and go back down **Barralton Hill,** and retrace the route to the start. The back side of Mitchell Hill is a pretty good practice hill, too.

Anyway, you get the picture. You could go all of the way around on 44, Weavers Run, Pauleys Gap and Pendleton and climb up Pendleton Road, too. There's a sign on it that says, "This Section Closed During Ice or Snow." I haven't even seen that on Pottershop. Pendleton is climbable, though.

So you really have several pretty good hills to think about –

Mitchell Hill, Knob Creek Road up the back side of Mitchell Hill, Barralton Hill Road, Pendleton Road up the other side of that hill, and Weavers Run Road up Cundiff Hill.

They're all combined with nice farm and residential roads that take you into and out of shady stretches of **Jefferson County Memorial Forest**. Where's the pain in that?

Spend a good part of the summer exploring the mathematical possibilities of this ride, and I promise you, Pottershop will give you no trouble come September.

Map Matters

This was one of two maps in the book that I found I could get a little larger within the page size if I tilted it so north is some direction other than straight up. The other one was the Audubon Dogwood Ride. They are both vaguely kidney-shaped, interestingly.

Route Sheet

0.0	Leave Welcome Center left on Mitchell Hill Road
1.0	Left at the top of Mitchell Hill
8.7	Right on KY 44
10.9	Right on Weavers Run Road
14.3	Right on Pendleton Road
21.0	Right on Blevins Gap Road
22.0	Right on Penile Road
23.5	Right on Manslick Road
23.8	Right on Keys Ferry Road
25.4	Right on Mitchell Hill Road
26.1	Back at Welcome Center

Huber Winery Ride

27 miles

Huber Winery
Start & End

Huber Rd.

St. John

Rd.

Engle Rd.

St. John

Hanka Rd.

Starlite Rd.

Scottsville Rd.

Skyline Dr. Rd.

Bethel-Frieberger

Banet

Knob

Moser

St. Mary Rd.

Skyline Dr.

Route follows gray line

Knob Rd.

Spickert

N

Huber Winery Ride

Twenty-seven miles. Several significant climbs. Start at Huber Winery, in Clark County, Ind., about 20 miles from downtown Louisville. Take I-64 from Louisville to the US 150-Greenville-Paoli exit. Take 150 to Navilleton Road, and follow the Huber Orchard signs.

My friend John Finley, who once worked in *The Courier-Journal's* New Albany news bureau, introduced me to the **Huber Winery** in the late 1970s. It was a delightful place—quiet, way out of the way, good food and drink. The wine was working away in the cellar beside the old barn, and it imparted a wonderful fresh smell that was just like taking the summer sunshine inside.

He staged a bike ride that started at U.S. 150 and Navilletown Road, a route that was then not too busy. It included a stop for lunch and a glass or two of wine, and a return to New Albany by St. Joseph Road.

St. Joe has a really steep, winding hill on it. Long story short, I crashed, ended up in the hospital and was the butt of a lot of jokes about wine and bicycling.

But I healed quickly and went back to Indiana's knobby hills soon, and have enjoyed riding there ever since. I just don't go down St. Joe Hill.

Hoosier Charm

The winery has grown some since then and added a few outbuildings, for ice cream, cheese and such. Its gift shop has moved up into the loft, and its vegetable and fruit offerings have expanded. There's a petting zoo now.

But it's still charming, and you will want to allow extra time to take it in at the beginning or end of your ride. Or both. You can pick strawberries or pumpkins in the correct season.

Head out down past the pond and left on St. John Road. Turn Right on Engle Road, and you soon find yourself at the **Joe Huber Farm and Restaurant.**

You will conclude that this is a ride you'll have to do several times to take in all of the area's offerings. Joe Huber is a cousin to the winery Hubers, and his place also offers all kinds of fresh vegetables and things to do. The restaurant offers first class country food.

Rolling, Twisting Country Roads

There are a lot of great country roads in the knobs, though, and it's mostly delightful to cycle. You should have a few 20 and 30 mile rides under your belt before you attempt this one. And bring your climbing legs.

Head south from Joe Huber's. Engle Road takes you to a piece of Scottsville Road, and you watch on the left for Hanka Road. You're going through farm country, though more and more strictly residential places are being built. Turn right on Starlite Road and left again on Bethel-Freiberger Road.

This is a heavily Catholic part of the county. You used to see the occasional bathtub Virgin here—a little shrine that takes advantage of the bandshell-like shape of an old-fashioned bathtub to honor St. Mary.

Turn right on Banet Road and right again on St. Mary's Road. Follow that around and down the hill, where you bear to the right in front of the church—**St. Mary of the Knobs Catholic Church**. It's a beautiful old church, and the stones in the graveyard out front bear some of the names you see on roads around here.

Climbing for a View

Continue down St. Mary and turn left on Spickert Knob Road. They don't call it that for nothing. We'll start climbing here, up to a group of roads that bear the name Skyline Drive here and there. On a clear day, if you can find a spot where there's a gap in the trees, you can see **downtown Louisville** from up here.

The fireworks of Kentucky Derby season's Thunder Over Louisville are quite a sight from up here, I have heard. Also, notice the **antenna farm**, with towers sprouting everywhere, serving many Louisville broadcasting stations.

Gear down and turn right onto Moser Knob Road—a very good practice hill, and just when you thought you were at a pretty good elevation already. You keep bearing left or turning left on Skyline Drive.

Besides nice views of Louisville and New Albany from up there, you will see a few houses you would like to live in. Pass Von Allman Road and turn left on St. John Road, and follow it around to Starlite. From there it's not far past the turnoff to Joe Huber's and a right turn back to the winery.

Route Sheet

0.0	Leave Parking Lot, Down past lake
0.4	Left on St. John Rd.
0.9	Right on Engle Rd.
1.2	Joe Huber's
3.0	Left on Scottsville
4.1	Left on Hanka
5.2	Right on Starlight
6.2	Left on Bethel-Freiberger
8.4	Right on Banet
8.5	Right on St. Mary's
9.9	Bear right in front of the Church
11.5	Left on Spickert Knob
12.1	Becomes S. Skyline Dr.
14.6	Right on Moser Knob
15.1	Bear left on N. Skyline
17.6	Left on N. Skyline
18.9	Pass Von Allman
19.7	Bear right
21.3	Left on St. John
25.9	Starlight
26.7	Right on Huber Road
27.2	Back at Huber's

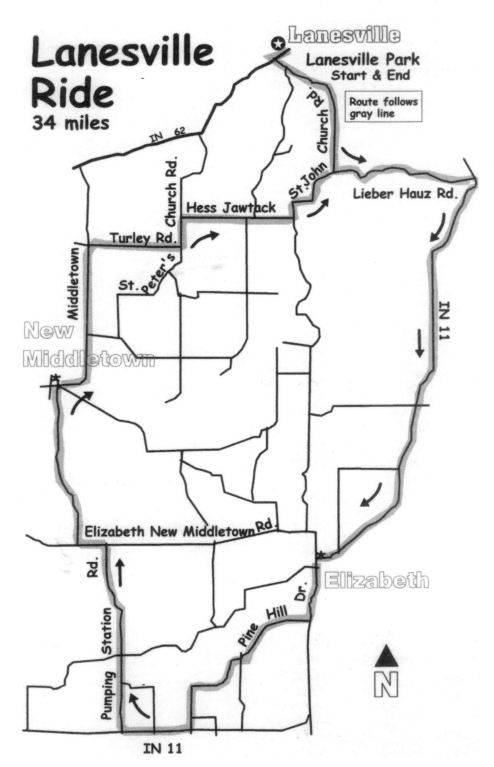

Lanesville Ride
34 miles

Lanesville

Lanesville Park
Start & End

Route follows
gray line

IN 62

St. John Church Rd.

Lieber Hauz Rd.

St. Peter's Church Rd.

Hess Jawtack

Turley Rd.

St. Peter's

Middletown

New Middletown

IN 11

Elizabeth New Middletown Rd.

Rd.

Pumping Station

Pine Hill Dr.

Elizabeth

N

IN 11

Lanesville Ride

> **Thirty-four miles. Very few hills. Start at Lanesville City Park, in Lanesville, Indiana, which is on IN 62, off I-64, about 12 miles west of Louisville. Go left off the I-64 ramp and left again onto IN 62 in Lanesville, then left on Park Road into the Park.**

This is a ride put together by Marilyn Motsch, she who finds rides without big hills. It is a very pleasant ride, taking advantage, in part—she told me—of roads Harrison County has paved because of the tax money it is receiving from the Caesar's Palace gambling boat.

And that's only fitting, because this ride, in a way, is a successor to the **Handy Andy Ride**, a long-time favorite of Louisville and Southern Indiana bike clubs that was essentially done in by the gambling boat.

The Handy Andy always started in New Albany, went up Edwardsville hill and out IN 11. It turned down IN 211 at the Handy Andy —a Laundromat that used to be at that corner—and returned to New Albany on IN 11, along the river.

Now there is a huge gambling complex on IN 111, and it's not as much fun to ride bikes along there anymore. So, as is more and more the case in the entire Louisville area, we have pushed our starting points for rides farther out into the countryside, and we ride where it's less crowded.

Old and New

Marilyn said she put this ride together from some old routes the clubs have taken, such as a wonderfully roller-coastery stretch of IN 11, and added some roads she found.

Once, she said, she was riding along there in the peaceful Indiana countryside, and she was charmed by the sight of a dove perched on a tombstone.

If you are doing this ride not too long after this book was published, you may still encounter Marilyn's mark at the corners—a stenciled hand with a pointing finger, telling you which way to turn.

A Slight Acclivity

Pedal out of the park and down IN 62 a ways, turn left on St. John's Church Road, and ride on out of town. You may notice that the road climbs just a little. But the ride is beautiful from the start, so you may not even notice.

And anyway, you're going to appreciate this stretch a lot, later. Turn left on the wonderfully-named Lieber Hauz road, and follow it out to IN 11, and turn right.

IN 11 is a road through beautiful Indiana farm country. I remember riding along here years ago when the Cold War was still underway, thinking it would be good to invite Russian cyclists on this ride because nobody who's ever seen it could bomb America.

Rollin', Rollin', Rollin'

There's a stretch of perfect roller coaster hills about seven miles into the ride. "Perfect" in the sense that, if you pedal down one side right, you get almost enough energy from the downhill to carry you up the uphill.

After about six miles on IN 11, or about 11 miles into the ride, you come to Indiana State Road 211, where there are a couple of stores if you need a stop. Both have soft drinks and sandwiches.

The **Elizabeth Mini Mart**, right on IN 11, is open 5 a.m. to 9 p.m. daily, and 8-9 Saturday. The 211 Food Mart, which is three tenths of a mile left on IN 211, has Sunday hours, 7 a.m. to 11 p.m., and a public restroom.

The 211 also is open from 6 a.m. to 11 p.m. weekdays, and 6 to midnight on Friday and Saturday.

Elizabeth

A bit more than a mile after IN 211, the route reaches **Elizabeth, Indiana**, a small town that also has store stops. IN 11 turns left at the end of town, and you turn with it.

You leave IN 11 outside of town to turn right onto Pine Hill Drive, but you catch up with 11 again three miles or so later, and take it right to Pumping Station Road.

That takes you up to Elizabeth-New Middletown Road, and into the little town of New Middletown—which is about 24 miles into the ride and usually calls for another stop.

Pie Time

For one thing, **The Lunch Box**, on the left at the one intersection that defines New Middleton, has great pie. And it is a charming gathering place. It calls itself a restaurant and Mini Mart, and says you can "Dine In" or "Carry Out" pizza, home-made pies or hot meals.

Area residents post notices there, such as "Lost Dog. Black and Tan coon hound. Lost at Pumping Station Road and Rogers Campground Road."

The proprietors have a sign that says, "No Pets in Store. Thank You. Tom & Mary." The Lunch Box is open 6 a.m. to 9 p.m. daily, including Saturday and Sunday.

Alternative

There's another place across the street called **Harpool's Grocery**, where they sell some hardware and motor oil along with snacks and groceries, and lottery tickets. It has soft drinks in an old-fashioned cooler that you access from the top.

Harpool's is closed on Sunday. "The Lord needed a day to rest, and so do we," said Barbara Harpool, who owns the store with her husband, Charles.

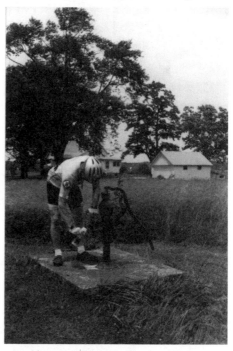

An old water pump on St. Peter's Church Road

Grave Matters

You leave New Middletown on Middletown Road, turning right between the two stores, and make a right on Turley Road. There's an **old graveyard** at the Turley Road corner. I have trouble resisting old graveyards.

You see those graves, some of people born in the 1700s, and wonder what their stories were. There is a man there born in Bergza, Kingdom of Bavaria, in 1805, and he died in 1860.

William Stine died at 22 in 1862, and you could cipher out an inscription on his stone if you worked at it:

> Our brother's left this world of woe
> for regions of eternal love
> 'twas God who called him from below
> to join in praising him above.

117

Sailing Home

Take Turley Road to a left on St. Peter's Church Road, and then a right on Hess Jawtack, and another left onto St. John's Church Road.

If you even noticed the slight hill coming up St. John's Church from the start you have forgotten it by now, and you are pleasantly surprised to go whizzing down the road for an effortless return to IN 62 and Lanesville Park.

"It's a good relatively short route," Marilyn said.

Route Sheet

0.0   Left on Indiana State Route 62 from Lanesville Park
0.3   Left on St. John's Church Road
2.7   Left on Lieber Hauz Road
5.1   Right on Indiana State Route 11
12.3   Left on IN 11 in Elizabeth
13.1   Right on Pine Hill Drive
16.3   Right on IN 11
17.5   Right on Pumping Station Road
20.6   Left on Elizabeth-New Middletown Road
23.7   Right on Middletown Road (at Lunch Box)
26.3   Right on Turley Road
27.8   Left on St. Peter's Church Road
28.1   Right on Hess Jawtack Road
29.9   Left on St. John's Church Road
33.5   Right on IN 62
33.7   Left to park

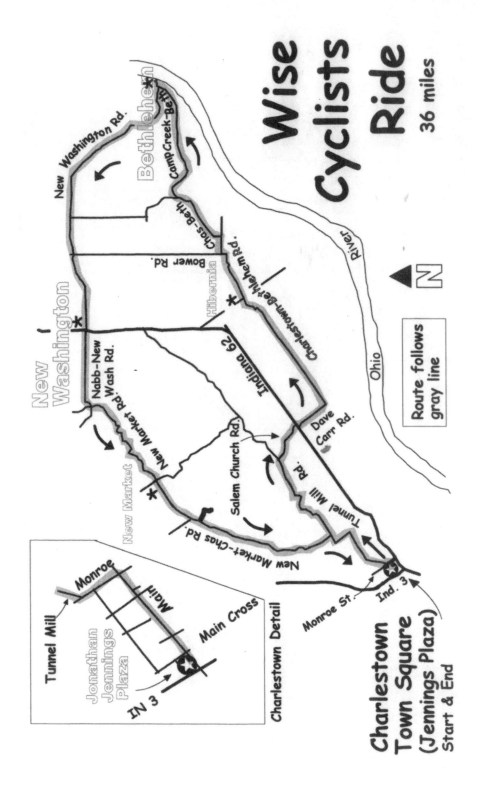

Wise Cyclists Ride
36 miles

N

Route follows gray line

New Washington Rd.
Bethlehem
Camp Creek-Beth.
Chas.-Beth.
Bower Rd.
Hibernia
Charlestown-Bethlehem Rd.
New Washington
Nabb-New Wash. Rd.
New Market Rd.
Indiana 62
Dave Carr Rd.
Salem Church Rd.
Tunnel Mill Rd.
New Market
New Market-Chas. Rd.
Ohio
River

Charlestown Detail

Tunnel Mill
Monroe
Jonathan Jennings Plaza
Main
Main Cross
IN 3

Monroe St.
Ind. 3

Charlestown Town Square
(Jennings Plaza)
Start & End

Wise Cyclists Ride

> **Thirty-six miles. Two big hills, and some smaller ones. Start at Jonathan Jennings Plaza, the town square, in Charlestown, Ind. It's on IN 62, about 14 miles from Louisville. To get to the square, take IN 3 left off of IN 62, and turn right at Main Street.**

This is a ride to Bethlehem that I used to take with two other *Courier-Journal* reporters—Martha Elson and Bill Pike—every year on a weekend between Thanksgiving and Christmas. We called ourselves "Three Wise Cyclists." It can get chilly most any weekend at that time of year there, so the ride is equipped with a few good hills to warm the body. There's nothing like a little exertion to generate body heat. But it's a good ride any time of year. You may sing as you ride—"O Little Town of Bethlehem," "We Three Kings," etc. Or not. After a few attempts, we generally didn't.

Charlestown

Take a left out of the square and go out Main Street to Monroe Street, and turn left again. Then turn right on Tunnel Mill Road.

Map Matters

To keep the route through Charlestown clear, while both keeping the rest of the route in perspective and keeping the map a manageable size for a stem clip, I had to put Charlestown detail in an inset.

Once you're on Tunnel Mill Road, your attention should go to the main map, until you're back on Monroe Street on the return trip.

> **Safety Note:** About three miles out you come to a steep downhill on Tunnel Mill. Be careful.

Lost Silver

As you ride along the bottomland at the foot of the hill you might keep an eye peeled for something shiny. Legend has it that Native Americans had a **silver mine** in this area someplace, with ore so plentiful that they made bullets out of it. The story is that a band of Indians blindfolded John Work—a miller whose home was just up the road—and took him to their mine. But he couldn't tell where he was, and though he searched the whole area for years afterward, he never found the place again.

Tunnel Mill

Work was a pioneer in these parts. He ran several mills for grinding grain, sawing wood and stone, and producing blasting powder. He also had a general store and a distillery. That's his **1811 Federal style house** on the left

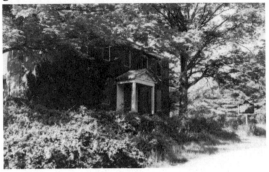

about three and a half miles out, behind the historic marker, all boarded up now.

Fourteen Mile Creek took a sharp bend around a stony promontory near here, and the miller blasted a tunnel through it to redirect the creek and get more power for his overshot wheels. He and a

John Work house

couple of helpers started tunneling in 1814 and it took them three years. John Work died in 1832, but his main mill lasted until 1927, when it burned.

You might ponder pioneer hardships as you climb the hill up past the **Tunnel Mill Boy Scout Reservation** about half a mile past Work's house. It's kind of steep and sort of long, but compared to blasting your way through a hill—using powder you made from saltpeter you gathered yourself—it's got to be a piece of cake.

Safety Note: After you turn right onto Salem Church Road about a mile past the scout camp, you'll negotiate a couple of little hills—heh—and reach Indiana 62. You jog right and then left. There often is quite a bit of traffic on that stretch of 62, and it moves fast. So be careful.

Hibernia

You take Dave Carr Road on the other side of 62, and then take a left onto the Charlestown-Bethlehem Road, which is sometimes abbreviated Chas-Beth, even on the road signs. Chas-Beth wanders around a bit, making right and left turns when you might least expect it. But it's well-signed.

About four miles from Dave Carr you come to the heart of the **Hibernia** community, centered where the road from Charlestown to Bethlehem crosses the road to **Boyer's Landing** on the Ohio River. Hibernia once had three general stores, a blacksmith and a barber, among other things.

Tender Coon

Lately, the town's claim to fame has been its annual **Coon Supper**, put on every March for 53 years by the **Owen Township Homemakers Club**. The supper's future was iffy as this book was being written, but Laveran Lorenz, club president, told me it did feature actual raccoon legs.

"There's not enough meat on the rest of them to bother with," she said. Mrs. Lorenz said she knows coon hunters who go out in November each year, and they'd save her the legs.

She'd clean them, soak them in salt water, and freeze them. In March, she'd thaw them, wash them again, roll them in seasoned flour, and fry them in oil. They'd go into an electric roaster at 10 a.m., and by the time the supper started at 4, the meat would be falling off the bone, she said.

Coon tastes kind of gamey, she said, like wild rabbit. "People say they've never eaten coon. But they try it and come back the following year," she said.

Ham, turkey, dressing, gravy, parsley potatoes, sweet potatoes, green beans, cake and pie are offered in addition to coon—all you can eat for $5 (a 2002 increase from $3.50). Still, Lorenz said, the crowd would take care of 60 to 70 coons.

Lorenz was 81 in 2002 and she said other stalwarts of the supper also were getting along in years. They were thinking of discontinuing it, but hadn't decided for sure.

Ride On

You'll know you're in **Hibernia** by the crossroads where Hibernia Road goes to the left and Blue Ridge Road goes right. You just ride straight on. Then you take a left on Boyer Road and a right back on good old Chas-Beth. A short distance later, Chas-Beth turns left.

Safety Note: About three miles after Hibernia the road takes a steep turn down Camp Creek Hill. It is steep and twisty, and sometimes on our November or early December trips down it, we found that road crews had spread cinders on it. Cinders help motor vehicles up icy roads, but when the ice is gone and the cinders remain, they can send skinny bicycle tires into a skid. So be careful.

Wild Turkeys

On the other hand, the countryside really starts to get wild and beautiful on this stretch. I once encountered a pair of wild turkeys here. They emerged from the brush on the left and eyed me warily, then sprinted down the road a ways and lifted off in a long, soaring hop back into the woods.

The Inn at Bethlehem

Near the bottom of the hill you turn right at a fork in the road and ride along delightful bottomland into **Bethlehem**. There used to be an **Inn** there, a bed and breakfast in an 1830 mansion facing the river. But the couple who restored it and operated it eventually gave it up, and the people who bought it wanted to live in it themselves. So there's no room at the inn anymore...that particular inn, anyway. There is another bed and breakfast around the corner and down the street, called **Storyteller's River House**. It's at 101 Bell St.

Bethlehem has been there since 1812, and was once a bustling river town. It was the most prominent of several landings on that stretch of the Ohio where farmers would meet the boats for store-bought things they needed, and bring wagonloads of grain, dressed hogs, produce and such to be shipped to city markets. Now it's mostly just a place where people have vacation houses, though some people live there year 'round and drive out to jobs.

Yuletide Postmark

The Bethlehem post office gets a lot of traffic just before Christmas, when people bring letters there for that Christmas-y postmark.

Most days, though, it doesn't take long to ride through the quiet streets of the entire town. On our fall rides my friends and I always took the steep drive down to the river bank and stood for awhile, watching boats, and examining flotsam and jetsam that had washed ashore.

But we learned that the nearest food and drink for travelers is in **New Washington**, about eight miles away, up a huge hill, so we seldom tarried long.

Big Hill. Huge Hill.

Non-cyclists who talk to you about your trip to Bethlehem won't believe you climbed the huge hill out of there. There actually are three ways to go, but they all have huge hills. The one that goes most directly to the food starts at the **old school**, which you will have passed on your way into town. Head away from the river.

Before you get to the hill though, notice the **town cemetery**, off to the right. It testifies to the town's more active past, because the tombstones are larger and more elaborate—and there are more of them— than you might expect from such a small town.

Then go ahead and climb the hill. It will not kill you. Put the old derailleur in stump-puller. Walking's not a crime, even. Think about what it must have been like to climb that thing in a provender-laden wagon. Or even to come down it with the entire year's output from your farm.

Fried Chicken

Follow the road from the top of the hill and you eventually get to **New Washington**. There's an outside soft drink machine at the hardware store, and you can get a sandwich, drinks and snacks at the **Corner Grocery** at Poplar and Main Streets. It's open on Sundays.

The wise cyclist contingent always went to **K-lyn's Kountry Kitchen**, a couple 10ths of a mile north on Indiana 62. I always got extra crispy fried chicken. You need calories to generate heat in November. At least that's what I said.

K-Lyn's was open only until 2 p.m. on Saturdays at this writing, and it was closed Sundays. There also is a small store in a **Marathon service station** on Ind. 62. It is open until 9 p.m. every day except Sunday, when it closes at 8 p.m.

New Market

You leave New Washington on the Nabb-New Washington Road, straight across Indiana 62 from the road you came in on. A couple of miles out, you turn left on New Market Road.

New Market is a crossroads town. Capt. Lewis C. Baird reported in his 1909 *History of Clark County* that market wagons on the way to the river from various directions used to rendezvous there. It's at the top of a hill, a pretty steep climb from three directions, and my guess is everybody had to rest.

Baird said the people from the farms started trading with the people headed back from the boats with their manufactured goods, and soon it was a market.

Baird said the place had three stores, a saloon, and a blacksmith shop in 1845, but was down to one store by 1909. Newspaper accounts say there were a couple of lively honky-tonks there in the early 20th century.

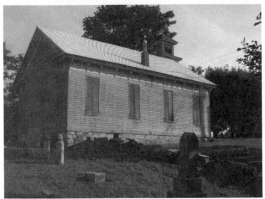

The Presbyterian Church in New Market

There's a picturesque old **Presbyterian church** in New Market, built in 1874 and moldering away since its congregation merged with others in 1978.

Go straight on through town, and head back toward Charlestown, through farmland and woods. Watch for a **Swiss-style chalet** on the right. I once saw a Bobwhite quail on this stretch, marching along the edge of the road with four or five miniatures of itself in a queue behind.

Turn right on Tunnel Mill, left on Monroe and right on Main, and you'll find yourself back at the square in **Charlestown**.

Route Sheet

0.0   Leave Charlestown town square on Main Street
0.4   Left on Monroe St.
0.5   Right on Tunnel Mill Road
3.2   Caution - twisty downhill
3.5   Tunnel Mill house
4.0   Pretty good climb
5.2   Right on Salem Church Road
6.3   Jog right across IN 62 onto Dave Carr Road
7.3   Left on Charlestown-Bethlehem Road
10.9   Hibernia
12.2   Left on Boyer Road
12.3   Right on Chas-Beth
12.8   Left on Chas-Beth
14.2   Caution - twisty downhill
14.8   Right on Chas-Beth
17.8   Bethlehem
17.8   Left (or right, if you've been
around town) on New
Washington Road
25.8   Cross IN 62 in New
Washington onto Nabb-New Washington Rd.
28.0   Left on New Market Road
33.3   Right on Tunnel Mill
35.2   Left on Monroe St.
35.3   Right on Main St.
35.7   Town Square

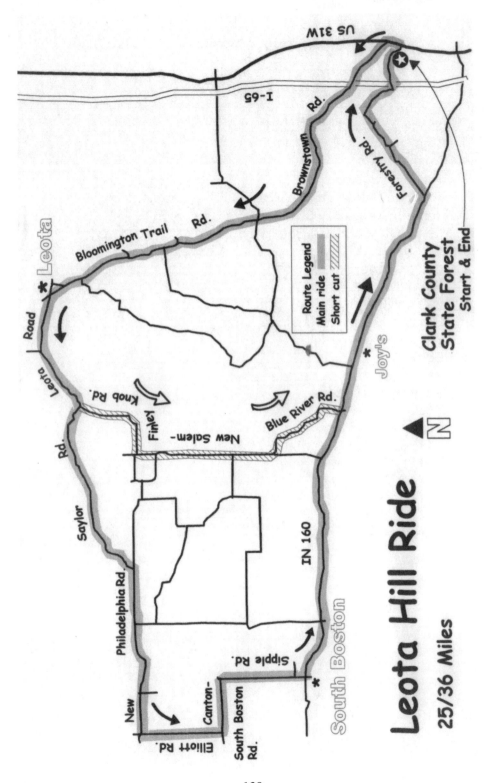

US 31W

I-65

Brownstown Rd.

Forestry Rd.

Leota

Bloomington Trail Rd.

Route Legend
Main ride
Short cut

Road

Leota

Rd.

Knob Rd.

Finley

New Salem-

Blue River Rd.

Joy's

Clark County
State Forest
Start & End

Saylor

N

Philadelphia Rd.

IN 160

New

Canton-

South Boston
Rd.

Sipple Rd.

South Boston

Elliott Rd.

Leota Hill Ride

25/36 Miles

128

Leota Hill Ride

Twenty-six or 36 miles. One big hill and some consecutive smaller hills, especially on the 36-mile route. Potential for some traffic on the return. Start at Clark County Forest, on US 31, about two miles north of Henryville, Ind., about 21 miles north of Louisville.

I think it is the melodious name of **Leota, Indiana,** that most attracts cyclists, though it sits at the junction of a couple of great cycling roads.

In any case, cyclists seem to love it, and my friend Alison Ewart said at least one Leota ride should be in this book.

The town existed for years as **Finley Crossroads,** named for John Finley, an early settler of the area. But Mathias Mount once owned a store there, and he applied for—and received—a postmaster's commission, and was given an opportunity to name the town.

He'd lost a daughter earlier to a childhood disease, and her name was Leota. She's buried in the churchyard at the **Old Ox Church,** not far off Bloomington Trail Road southeast of the town.

Daffodil Lady

That information comes from Helen Trueblood, a woman of advanced youth who is an authority both on daffodils and on **Finley Township,** where Leota is situated, among other things.

She doesn't tell her age, she said, because her mother said a lady does not do that. But she remembers well things that happened in Leota 70 and more years ago.

She lives on the hill just above the barn that faces Leota's **landmark covered bridge.** She hosts daffodil shows there, sanctioned by the American Daffodil Society, and even has had one national convention.

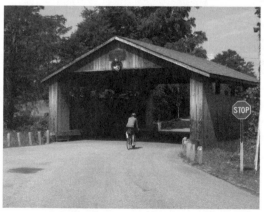

Leota's covered bridge

Old Roads

Leota lies at the intersection of Bloomington Trail Road, which carried pioneer traffic from Louisville through Bloomington to Indianapolis, and Leota Road.

The latter, Mrs. Trueblood said, is a section of the old **Cincinnati Trace**, surveyed between 1799 and 1805.

The roads come together right where both cross **Cooney Creek**, under a covered bridge, which dates just to 1995. There was an old concrete bridge at the crossroads, Mrs. Trueblood said, and it was losing ground to heavy farm loads that crossed it. The county wanted to replace it with a couple of large sewer tiles.

But townspeople prevailed on a man with experience building decorative covered bridges in parks to build that instead. It's more in keeping with Leota's flavor and heritage, but it keeps Mrs. Trueblood busy watching so that "some knothead" with a high load doesn't come through and tear it up. That has only happened once, so far.

Forest Start

The ride starts at the entrance to the **Clark County Forest**, with a left turn onto US 31, and another left onto Brownstown Road three tenths of a mile up the road.

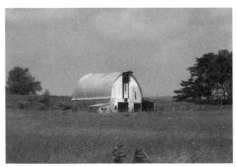

Brownstown becomes Bloomington Trail Road where it passes from Clark into **Scott County** about three and a half miles from the ride's start. There are scenic farmsteads and old graveyards worth exploring all the way on up **Bloomington Trail**.

There's an old church to the right where Ox Road comes in, about seven miles up, and little **Leota Mount** is buried there. Ox Road was named for **Old Ox**, the chief of an Indian band that used to camp near Vienna and trade with early settlers.

Scenery along Bloomington Trail

Spring Tonic

Schoolhouse Road takes off to the right just above Leota and connects with Leota Road coming in from Vienna. The route stays straight. Mrs. Trueblood was a pupil in the school that used to be there, the year she got whooping cough so bad her father thought he was going to have to take her to Arizona to recover.

But John R. Ritchie suggested a little of his spring tonic, and that cleared it right up. Made her grow to nearly adult height, too, she said.

"John R. would get in the woods and gather different things, and then he would get something from New York. He'd mix it all up and boil it and strain it," Mrs. Trueblood said.

Then Mrs. Trueblood's father, who hauled chickens and other farm goods to the haymarket in Louisville, would bring back alcohol, which Ritchie used to give his potion just the right medicinal quality.

John R. is not to be confused with Dr. John Ritchie, one of Scott County's first doctors, and Mrs. Trueblood's great-great grandfather.

Bucktown

You ride through the Leota bridge and take Leota Road to the left. But take note that when you cross the bridge, you leave Leota and enter a suburb, called **Bucktown**.

Even though it's a subordinate part of the community, Bucktown takes part in the **Leota Frolic**, held every year on the fourth weekend in August, with things to eat, flea market items to buy, music, and various kinds of contests. A lot of the parking is over there.

Aside from the Frolic, though, there is no longer any commercial activity in Leota, though the last of a series of stores still stands near the bridge, and is opened as a museum for Frolic.

Finley Knob Hill

As you ride up Leota Road toward the hills, notice that one of the creek bottoms you pass is deeper than you expect and has a sort of a gouged look. Mrs. Trueblood said that is because heavy rains really send water pouring off those knobs.

That's **Finley Knob** just ahead, and, surprise, that's really **Finley Knob Hill** you are about to climb. I wanted to get both the name, Leota, and the hill in the ride title, without making it too long.

It's a significant hill. Better put her in stump-puller. If you've got a third chain wheel, go to that. If not, it's still doable. Just grind away.

Decisions, Decisions

There's a great view from the top, where you face a choice. You can take Saylor Road to the right and make this a 36-mile ride, or you can take New Salem-Finley Knob Road to the left and hold your mileage to about 26.

The 36-mile version is a bit hillier, but there are no more Finley Knobs to worry about.

It's a tough choice in a way, because if you turn left you will miss **New Philadelphia**, and if you turn right you will miss **New Salem**.

But don't agonize too much. Dave Runge and I turned right and we *still* missed New Philadelphia, and didn't find out where it was until we got to South Boston and asked. Then we rode up to New Salem, and only found *it* by paying strict attention.

Whiskey Stories

For the record, New Philadelphia is just after the point where Leval Ratt Road comes into the route from the right. There is a home in a former school house there.

I read in an 1884 history at the Filson Historical Society library that "a man named Sisson" started a saloon in New Philadelphia once, and learned that it was not a saloon kind of town. Townspeople broke in one night and stove in all of his barrel heads, and let the liquor pour into the streets. There never was a saloon there again, the history said.

But before you get to New Philadelphia, still on Saylor Road, at about mile 12.3, a Whiskey Hollow Road takes off to the left. There must be some stories in that.

"About every little settlement around Leota had somebody who made moonshine," Mrs. Trueblood said. "That was their antiseptic. Alcohol kills germs."

Rollers

You take Saylor Road down to New Philadelphia Road, turn right and proceed through the town itself, then turn left on Elliott Road. You will notice along here that the roads have begun taking an up and down attitude, rolling down one hill and up the next.

None of the hills are particularly big, but the relentlessness with which one follows the other gives you some good hill practice.

Mauck's General Store

You turn left from Elliott Road onto Canton-South Boston Road, which takes a right after a while and becomes Sipple Road. Roll down that last hill, cross the Middle Fork of the Blue River, and you'll find yourself at Indiana State Route 160, South Boston, and **Mauck's General Store.**

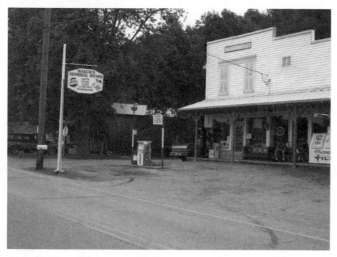
Mauck's General Store

Mauck's advertises the "Best Pizza in Town," and you have to agree. Because a quick glance around tells you that unless you have a lunch invitation to a private home, it's the *only* pizza in town.

Mauck's offers lunchmeat sandwiches from the meat case, though, and plate lunches, along with all sorts of soft drinks, and gifts. There are tables where you can sit to eat. There is a pot-bellied stove, and there are a lot of friendly people, some of them playing cards.

It's open from 6 a.m. to 6:30 p.m. Monday through Friday, and from 7:30 a.m. to 5 p.m. on Saturday. It's closed on Sunday.

Safety Note: The route heads back toward the forest on IN 160 from South Boston. It's the main road from Charlestown through Henryville to Salem, and it can get busy at times. I've never found traffic too oppressive, but be careful. And if you're in a group, ride single file when traffic builds up behind you.

Joy's Quick Stop

If you have taken the 26-mile version of the ride, you won't get as far as Mauck's at South Boston. Your route comes out on 160 about five miles east of there.

But about a mile farther east—six or so miles from Mauck's, for you long riders—you come to **Joy's Quick Stop**, which also offers sandwiches, pizza and soft drinks, and it's open on Sunday.

Hours at Joy's are 8 a.m. to 6:30 p.m. Monday through Saturday, and 8-2 on Sunday.

Cyclist's Privilege

Follow IN 160 east to Forestry Road, about four miles past Joy's, and turn left. The road passes some farms and gets into woods. About a mile along it, you'll see a gravel road going to the left, to a barricade.

That's to keep cars from entering the state forest there, but not you. Walk your bike, if you need to, the 60 or 70 yards around the barricade, then remount and turn right on the asphalt road in the forest.

Bear left and then right and cross high above I-65, and you'll find yourself back at the forest parking lot.

Route Sheets

0.0	Leave Henryville State Forest entrance parking lot, left on US 31
0.4	Left on Brownstown Road (becomes Bloomington Trail Road)
8.9	Leota. Left out of bridge on Leota Road
10.8	Start Big Hill
11.3	Right on Saylor Road at top of Hill
14.9	Right on New Philadelphia Road .
16.3	New Philadelphia (where Leval Ratt Road comes in)
17.9	Left on Elliott Road
19.3	Left on Canton-South Boston Road
20.3	Right on Sipple Road
21.6	Mauck's Store, South Boston, Left on IN 160
27.7	Joy's Quick Stop
32.0	Left on Forestry Road
33.2	Left through barricade, right on the forest road
33.5	Bear left

33.7	Bear right
35.6	Back at parking lot

Short Version

0.0	Leave Henryville State Forest Entrance parking lot, left on US 31
0.4	Left on Brownstown Road (becomes Bloomington Trail Road)
8.9	Leota. Left out of bridge on Leota Road
10.8	Start Big Hill
11.3	Left on New Salem-Finley Knob Road at top of Hill
13.8	New Salem
15.9	Left on Blue River Road
17.7	Left on IN 160
18.8	Joy's Quick Stop
23.1	Left on Forestry Road
24.2	Left through barricade, right on the forest road
24.5	Bear left
24.7	Bear right
26.4	Back at parking lot

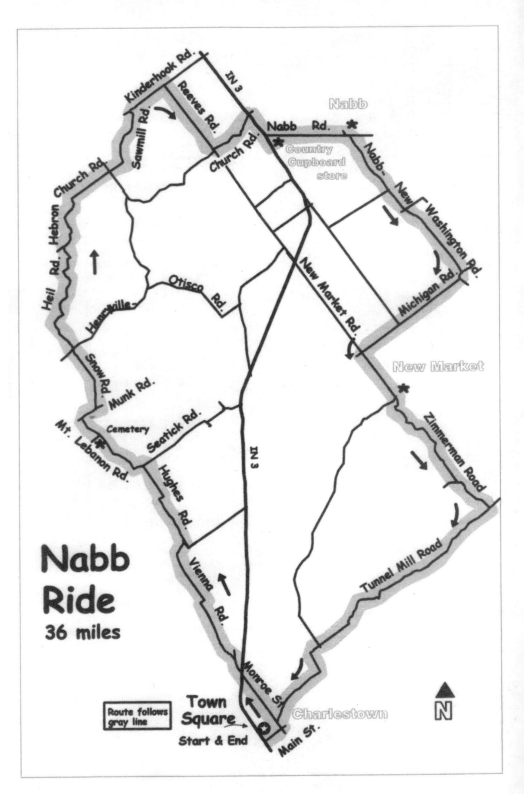

Nabb
Ride
36 miles

Route follows
gray line

Town
Square
Start & End

N

Nabb Ride

Thirty-Six miles. Hilly in spots, with one big hill just before the end. Start at Jonathan Jennings Plaza, the Charlestown town square. Charlestown in on IN 62, about 14 miles northeast of Louisville, and the square is on Main Street, just off IN 3.

This is another ride that shows what good riding there is in the Indiana counties close to Louisville, and also how fast it could disappear. There are a lot of houses under construction out there.

The ride also illustrates that there are a lot of stories on the road, if you take time to find out about them. I found one on Mt. Lebanon Road that I'm not sure I wanted to know about, but that everybody probably should know about. But first let me get you on the road.

Leaving Charlestown

Leave **Jennings Plaza** to the left, out Main Street to a left on Monroe Street. **Jonathan Jennings**, incidentally, was a lawyer who settled in **Charlestown** in 1809, became an Indiana territory delegate to Congress, helped Indiana become a state and served as its first governor, and later served several terms as an Indiana congressman. He's buried nearby.

Cross Indiana State Route 3 onto Edgewood Drive, and watch for Vienna Road to fork off to the left. Take that left fork, and then, a mile or so up the road, jog right on a chunk of Jack Temple Road and continue on Vienna Road.

Turn left onto Harry Hughes Road. The road itself turns left a bit more than a mile later—right where Seatick Road comes in from the right—and becomes Mt. Lebanon Road. A little more than a mile after that, you come to **Mt. Lebanon Presbyterian Church**, which has an old cemetery.

The Park Murders

An 1871 tombstone there has this intriguing inscription: "This monument to Cyrus M. Park and family is erected as a memorial to their tragic deaths caused by an axe in the hands of avaricious assassins."

Besides Cyrus, who was 44 when he died, the stone names his wife, Isabella, 41; their son, John, 10, and their daughter, Helen, 14. They died Nov. 11, except for Helen, who lingered until Dec. 8.

I asked a couple of people I encountered along the road about the incident, but nobody knew anything. So eventually I looked in *Courier-Journal* microfilm.

It was a horrendous story of murder in the night, told in considerable gory detail by a *Courier-Journal* reporter who visited the Park cabin, which was very near the cemetery. The aftermath of the crime was just as bad, in many respects. Because family clothes were taken, the story said, officials concluded that the murders must have been committed by "Negroes" —even though there was some indication Park had white enemies connected with disagreements over construction of the Mt. Lebanon Church.

Investigators on Horseback

A number of black men were rounded up immediately, the newspaper said, and a confession was forced from one who seemed shaky on his whereabouts on the murder night. The story said neighbors got him to implicate two other men and himself, by taking him into the woods at night and threatening to kill him.

He later told a reporter that none of it was true. He said he made it up rather than be killed on the spot, and that he had wavered on his whereabouts because he was married and with another woman.

Anyway, he and the other two men were taken to jail in Charlestown, and citizens of the community went looking for evidence against them.

"Night and day horsemen scoured the county—visiting every hill, valley or ravine, every habitation of man or beast, overhauling, turning topsy-turvy, ransacking every imaginable nook or corner that might by the barest possibility be the hiding place of even the faintest trace that might lead ultimately to the detection of the perpetrators of the foul and brutal deed," the paper said.

I assume that was not much fun for those searched, especially the black families.

Lynching

Anyway, any evidence they found apparently was not very convincing, because a grand jury then in session adjourned five days later without returning an indictment. It was not to reconvene for two weeks.

Five days after the original crime was discovered, men in masks broke the suspects out of jail and hanged them in the woods. The victim's names were George Johnson, Squire Taylor and Charles Davis.

A *Courier-Journal* reporter, anticipating the lynching, was in the jail when the mob arrived, and he described a three-hour effort to break the men out with large hammers and chisels, in menacing and then horrifying detail.

The account referred to the hangmen as "Ku Kluxers," and said the leader's mask was loose enough that his face could be seen occasionally. He "resembled very much Andrew Stone of Charlestown," the story said. "But it was not him."

No Real Resolution

I found one mention of the incident in an informal Clark County history at the Jeffersonville library. But it said only that citizens had taken the law into their own hands. It didn't say whether it was ever learned if the men were really guilty. Thelma Masters, a 100-year-old citizen of Henryville, told me the crime was still a topic of conversation when she came to town as a little girl in 1910, but she hadn't heard anything about it for many years.

The Route Continues

Anyway, maybe sometimes you need to be careful what you ask. Continue on past the church, taking a right on Munk Road, a left on Snow Road, and another left on Zollman-Snow Road.

There's a bit of a downhill as you approach Henryville-Otisco road, which you cross onto Heil Road. Heil is a very nice stretch of country riding, with some sweeping views of rolling bottomland along Silver Creek.

But just when you think you've left civilization behind, you come up on Deer Run Drive and a big new subdivision on the left. Stay on Heil Road, though, and take it to a right on Hebron Church Road.

Sights to See

You'll pass a **covered bridge** along there—a new one, with sylvan-looking pastures and white fence beyond it. I'll tell you more about that on the next ride, Marysville. Same for the elk ranch you'll notice on the left a bit farther on.

Hebron Church eventually tees in to a road that's been named Beagle Club Road to the left, and Dieterlan Road to the right. Jog right on Dieterlan, and take a quick left on Sawmill Road.

There's a pasture full of **miniature horses** about a half-mile later on Sawmill. Almost a mile later, you find the road's name has changed to Slate Ford Road, and you turn right on Kinderhook Road.

Watch for Reeves Road on the right and take it southeast, over a series of rollers that will give you some practice in building momentum downhill to carry you part of the way up the next hill.

Turn left on Church Road, which will take you one mile over to IN 3. And in that mile, Church Road's name changes to County Line Road and then Stucker Road.

Buy Stuff

Turn right on IN 3 and ride half a mile to **Kristin's Country Cupboard**. I used to stop there a lot with a group of teenage bike riders that once was attached to the Louisville Club. We'd get soft drinks and sandwiches from the meat case, and rest.

As this book was written, the store had been spruced up a bit since those days, and had booths for sit-down dining. It is open from 6 a.m. to 9 p.m. Monday through Saturday, and 6 to 8 on Sunday.

Backtrack up IN 3 about a tenth of a mile and turn right on IN 362, also known as Nabb Road, also known as County Line Road. There are antique cars and car parts, and a great antique store in **Nabb**.

When you're done looking around, turn right on Nabb-New Washington Road.

RAGBRAI?

If you've ever been on the Register's Annual Great Bicycle Ride Across Iowa, the next series of roads will make you nostalgic. Or if you haven't, they'll be good practice in case you ever want to go. They go straight for a ways, then turn 90 degrees, and then go straight again, just like in Iowa.

Anyway, turn right on Harry Bauer Road, and almost immediately right again on Michigan Road. Check out the **Buckminster Fuller geodesic dome house** over to the left. After awhile, turn left on New Market Road and cruise into **New Market**.

Beyond New Market you leave Iowa behind. The road actually curves. You cross **Fourteen Mile Creek** south of town and then take a delightful trek along **Polk Run**, a tributary that has rural Indiana written all over it.

New Market Road becomes Zimmerman Road along there at some point, and leads you to a right turn on Tunnel Mill Road. Follow it down the hill past the **Boy Scout camp** and the **old miller's house**.

Practice Hill

And then, just when you thought I'd managed to find you a ride without a significant hill, there it is. You look up and think, "Oh no." But it won't kill you. Just put it in stump puller, and grind your way on up.

Then ride on in to Monroe Street, hang a left, turn right on Main Street, go four tenths of a mile, and there you are.

Route Sheet

0.0	Leave square on Main
0.3	Left on Monroe Street
1.7	Cross IN 3 onto Edgewood Dr.
1.9	Left onto Vienna Road
3.1	Jog right on a chunk of Jack Temple Road, continue on Vienna
4.5	Left on Harry Hughes Road
6.1	Left on Mt. Lebanon Road, where Seatick Road comes from right
7.3	Mt. Lebanon Presbyterian Church and cemetery, straight on Mt. Lebanon
7.7	Right on Munk Road
8.0	Left on Snow
8.5	Left on Zollman-Snow Road
9.3	Cross Henryville-Otisco Road, onto Heil Road
11.4	Right onto Hebron Church Road
11.6	Covered Bridge on right
13.5	Jog right on Dieterlen and go straight on Sawmill
14.8	Right onto Kinderhook Road
15.5	Right onto Reeves Road
16.9	Left on Church Road
17.9	Right on IN 3
18.5	Kristin's Country Cupboard. Backtrack up IN 3, right on IN 362, Nabb Road
20.1	Nabb. Right on Nabb-New Washington Road
23.4	Right on Harry Bauer Road
23.5	Right on Michigan Road, Dome on left
25.9	Left on New Market Road
26.9	New Market. Straight on New Market Road, which becomes Zimmerman Road
29.8	Right on Tunnel Mill Road
33.0	Big hill
35.7	Left on Monroe Street
35.8	Right on Main Street
36.2	End at town square

Marysville Meander
39/23 miles

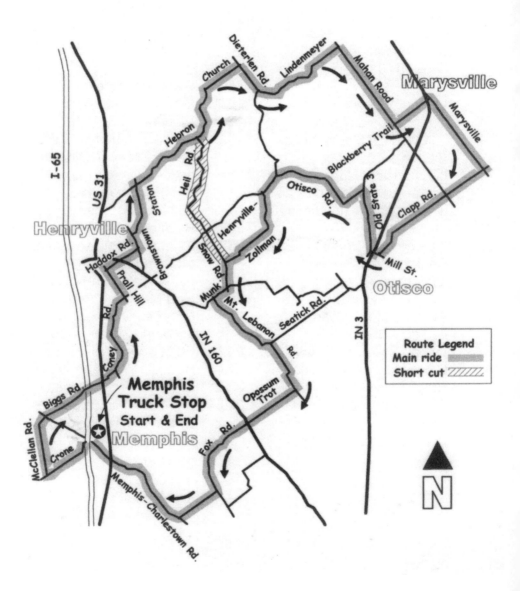

Marysville Meander

Thirty-nine or 23 miles. Some hills, but no big ones. Start at the Country Style Plaza truck stop, on the right side of I-65, about 16 miles north of Louisville.

The **Louisville Bicycle Club** used to gather for rides on about every Saturday and Sunday. But it grew, and attracted members with working days that varied, and now it has a ride about every day, at least in summer.

Some of the days have taken on personalities of their own. The Wednesday morning group, for example, tends to be old timers—including retired folks—and people who ride with them.

They like to stop and smell the roses. Or order meals at restaurants. They do not get in a hurry. They are my kind of riders. This ride was inspired by one of theirs, and it starts at a frequent starting place for the Wednesday morning group—the **Country Style Plaza.**

Wander Up to Henryville

Take a right out of the parking lot onto Memphis-Blue Lick Road, go under I-65 and turn left immediately on Crone Road. Turn right on McClellan Road and cross Memphis-Blue Lick Road again, to find yourself on Biggs Road.

Follow Biggs under I-65 again and across US 31, where it becomes Caney Road. Take that up to Prall Hill Road. Make a left there and check to see if **Donnie Guthrie's buffalo** are out and about. They should be on the left. Notice his **horse-drawn omnibus**, also.

Prall Hill goes most of the way into **Henryville**, and if you were with the Wednesday morning group, they'd probably ride on up and take a right on Pennsylvania Street and then a left on IN 160. They'd follow that to **Schuler's Family Restaurant**, out by I-65, and get a piece of pie or an omlette.

Schuler's is open 6 a.m. to 9 p.m., seven days a week.

Head for the Countryside

But this route turns left just short of Pennsylvania Street, on Haddox Road, and goes up a bit of a hill. It crosses IN 160 onto Castetter Road, passes some houses of the kind that often cause my friend David Runge to say, "I could live here," and turns left on Brownstown Road.

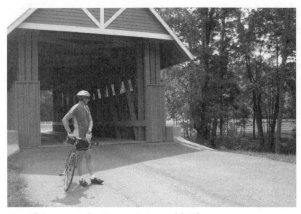

David Runge at the Garman's covered bridge

Very shortly, it turns right on Staton Road, and takes that a mile or so to a right on Hebron Church Road. There's another bit of a hill out there a ways.

That **covered bridge** on the right about 10 miles out is part of a retreat center being developed by Charles and Phyllis Garman of New Albany. Beyond the bridge are green pastures behind white fences, and tree-covered hills. I saw a couple of deer dash out of the meadow and into the trees once when I was riding by.

Leaving the World Behind

Mrs. Garman said the bridge, which she and her husband had built, it is a sort of symbolic portal. Business and other groups come to the site for day conventions. "We wanted to give the feeling that you are leaving the busy world, that we're taking you out of the hurried, scurried world," she said.

Eventually they will have sleeping lodges there for weekend retreats. The bridge is a small one by 19th century standards, but Mrs. Gorman said it's built strong enough to carry Greyhound buses, fire trucks and semi-trailers.

Elk and Red Stags

A bit farther up Hebron Church Road, on the left, is the **White Oak Elk Ranch,** owned by Rick Davis, who also is one of the owners of **Davis Brothers Travel Plazas.** Davis said he has some 1,100-pound bull elk in there, along with some fallow deer from Europe and some white tail deer. He also has some red stags, which are European elk. He raises breeding stock and does some hunting there, bringing friends in to a 1935 barn remodeled into a lodge.

"I go up there for R and R more than anything," Davis said. "It's a real pleasant place."

Dog Talk

A bit further along Hebron Church Road one day, David Runge and I met a woman named Toni Shake, who was out working on her grass with her

144

dog, Callie, and who agreed to look up the phone number of somebody she thought would know about the covered bridge.

Then she asked us all about cycling, and wondered in particular what we do when dogs chase us. She suggested it might be a good idea to quote scripture to them, which I had to say was something I hadn't tried.

In fact, I don't know much scripture. But I came across this: "A righteous man has regard for the life of his beast." Proverbs 12:10. I could maybe shout that and then add, "But don't push it!"

On to Marysville

Hebron Church Road eventually tees into Dieterlen Road, where you hang a right and then bear left up a little hill onto LindenMayer Road. I saw

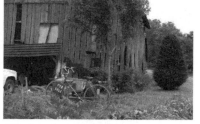

a **native American tipi** along LindenMayer road once.

Turn Right on Mahan Road and left on Blackberry Trail, and then cross Indiana State Route 3 into **Marysville**. There's not much there, really. Marysville is an old railroad town that according to history books never really took off.

Bike for sale on Mahan Road

You can get soft drinks from machines in front of a hardware store on IN 3, but there's more provender five miles ahead.

Otisco

Turn right on Marysville Road and follow it out to Clapp Road and another right. Ride that down to Mill Street in Otisco, and take that right across IN 3 to the **H&B Grocery**. The Wednesday morning people like the H&B, too.

You can get soft drinks there, and all kinds of snacks, and sandwiches out of the meat case, and even fried chicken. It's open from 5:30 a.m. to 9 p.m. Monday through Thursday, 5:30 to 10 Friday and Saturday, and 8 a.m. to 9 p.m. on Sunday.

Turn right on Old State 3 behind the store, and then a left on Henryville-Otisco Road about a mile out.

Mt. Moriah and The Colonel

A couple of miles along Henryville-Otisco, watch for **Mt. Moriah Church** and its attendant cemetery. I noticed that the church looked much newer than the cemetery, and asked about it in Henryville.

Butch Furnish and Thelma Masters said the church burned awhile back, when the **Clegg School** across the road caught fire, and **Col. Harland Sanders**, of Kentucky Fried Chicken fame, helped rebuild it.

"Col. Sanders was a Clegg," Mrs. Masters said. She turned 100 in September, 2001, and knows quite a lot about Henryville and area. The Cleggs apparently are on Sanders' mother's side.

Anyway, the Colonel's parents—Wilbert D. Sanders, who died in 1895, and Margaret Ann Sanders, who died in 1935—are buried in the cemetery by the church.

Zollman Road

A short distance past the church you take a left on Zollman Road, up a little hill, and cut across a couple of miles to Snow Road. Somewhere along there—about halfway across, Furnish said—**Col. Sanders** was born, in a house that's no longer there.

Col. Sanders himself is buried in Cave Hill Cemetery in Louisville. There's a yellow line painted on the pavement from one of the entrances to his grave, because it's the most asked-for grave in the cemetery. So now you're among those who know where his parents are buried.

Turn left at the end of Zollman Road onto Snow Road, and then right on Munk Road, and left on Mt. Lebanon Road. Take that down to Opossum Trot—a road I knew I had to ride as soon as I saw its name—and follow that across IN 160 to Fox Road.

Turn with Fox past Whittinghill Road, and take a right on Charlestown-Memphis Road. That takes you through Memphis across US 31, and back to the truck stop.

Alternatives

If you want to make this a 23-mile ride instead of a 36-mile one, there's a good shortcut. Just take a right on Heil Road, about 10 miles from the start. You get a nice stretch there through scenic farmland along **Silver Creek**.

But you miss the covered bridge, the elk farm, possibly the tipi (if it's still there), Marysville, Otisco, and the graves of Col. Sanders' parents. And you have to climb a bigger hill than any other on the ride, on Snow Road just past Henryville-Otisco Road. It hardly seems worth it. But you know how far you want to ride.

Route Sheet

0.0	Leave parking lot, Country Style Plaza truck stop
0.4	Left on Crone Road
1.6	Right on McClellan Road
2.8	Cross Memphis-Blue Lick Road onto Biggs Road
4.1	Cross US 31W onto Caney Road
6.1	Left on Prall Hill Road
6.7	Right on Haddox Road (Hill)
7.1	Cross 160 onto Castetter Road
7.5	Left on Brownstown Road
7.8	Right on Staton Road
8.9	Right on Hebron Church Rd
10.6	Covered Bridge on Right
13.1	Right on Dieterlen Road
13.7	Bear left on LindenMayer Road, Dieterlen goes right
15.7	Right on Mahan Road
17.6	Left on Blackberry Trail
18.4	Cross IN 3 into Marysville
18.5	Right on Marysville Road
20.2	Right on Clapp Road
23.0	Right on Mill Street, Cross IN 3 to store
23.2	Right on Old State 3
24.5	Left on Henryville-Otisco Rd
26.8	Mt. Moriah Church and Cemetery
27.1	Left on Zollman Road
29.1	Left on Snow Road
29.5	Right on Munk Road
29.8	Left on Mt. Lebanon Road
32.5	Right on Opossum Trot Rd
33.7	Cross IN 160 onto Fox Rd
35.5	Fox turns past Whittinghill Road, turn with Fox
36.4	Right onto Charlestown-Memphis Road
38.3	Cross US 31 W
38.9	Back at start

Short Cut Alternative

0.0	Leave parking lot, Country Style Plaza truck stop
0.4	Left on Crone Road
1.6	Right on McClellan Road
2.8	Cross Memphis-Blue Lick Road onto Biggs Road
4.1	Cross US 31W onto Caney Road
6.1	Left on Prall Hill Road
6.7	Right on Haddox Road (Hill)
7.1	Cross 160 onto Castetter Road
7.5	Left on Brownstown Road
7.8	Right on Staton Road
8.9	Right on Hebron Church Road
10.4	Right on Heil Road
12.5	Cross Henryville-Otisco Road onto Snow Road, up the hill
13.8	Right on Munk Road
14.1	Left on Mt. Lebanon Road
16.8	Right on Opossum Trot Road
18.0	Cross IN 160 onto Fox Road
19.8	Fox turns past Whittinghill Road, turn with Fox
20.7	Right onto Charlestown-Memphis Road
22.6	Cross US 31 W
23.2	Back at start

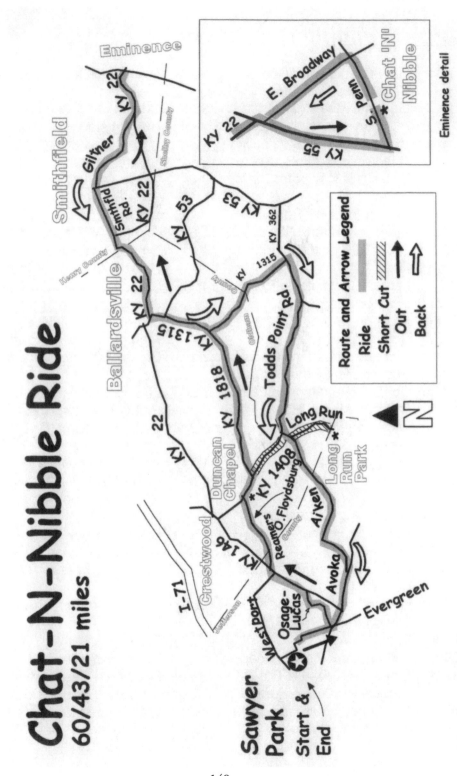

Chat-N-Nibble Ride
60/43/21 miles

Eminence

Smithfield

KY 22

Giltner

Shelby County

Smthfld Rd.

KY 22

KY 53

KY 53

KY 362

Henry County

Ballardsville

KY 22

KY 1315

KY 1315

KY 1818

Duncan Chapel

KY 22

Crestwood

I-71

KY 146

Osage-Lucas

Westport

Jefferson County

Evergreen

Avoka

Aiken

*KY 1408

Reamers Rd

O. Floydsburg

Oldham County

Todds Point Rd.

KY 1315

KY
1315

Oldham

Long Run

*

Long Run Park

Sawyer Park

Start & End

N

Eminence detail

E. Broadway

KY 22

KY 55

Penn

S.

* Chat "N" Nibble

Route and Arrow Legend

Ride

Short Cut

Out

Back

148

Chat-N-Nibble Ride

Sixty miles, 43 miles, or 21 miles. Small to moderate hills. Start at Tom Sawyer Park, off Westport Road, three quarters of a mile toward town from the Gene Snyder Freeway.

The Chat-N-Nibble is a good independence ride for those who've done those rides in the 'teens and '20s and might be feeling their oats.

It also has options for people still working up to that, or who don't have time on a particular day for a longer ride.

I offer three choices here. Well, five, actually. You can start at **E.P. Tom Sawyer State Park** and go for the full 60. Or you can miss some good countryside going and coming, and start from **Long Run Park** for about 42.

Or, you can take a short cut on Todds Point-Aiken Road and just head back for Sawyer from the KY 1408 and KY 362 intersection, for about 21 miles. They're all nice rides.

As I said at the beginning of the book, you can make your own options on any of these rides. If you just wanted a short ride and a nice smoked pork tenderloin sandwich with Alice Ferguson's special sauce, for example, you could just start at the church in Ballardsville for a 20-mile round trip.

Or you could stay on KY 22 past Eminence all of the way to Gratz, for 100 miles or so.

But first, the Chat-N-Nibble ride itself.

Map Matters

It's actually easy enough to find the **Chat-N-Nibble restaurant** once you arrive in **Eminence** on KY 22. But just in case you find it confusing, I enlarged the portion of the map showing that detail a little so you can get straight to the homemade pie. It's all part of the service.

Gratz Century

Years ago, my friend David Runge—now retired from a long-time job as an art teacher at New Albany High School—took a three-day camping ride with me up through Madison, Ind., Carrollton and Frankfort, Ky., and back to Louisville. I wrote about it for the *Courier-Journal* magazine, and David took the pictures.

He already was sort of a pathfinder for the Louisville bicycle club, famous then as now for "Runge Roads," which often are obscure, possibly steep, and not overly-paved. But they're guaranteed scenic. He won't use the words "rough," or "bumpy," preferring to say a road "has texture."

Anyway, he fell in love with the little town of **Gratz**, which is on a hill on the east side of the Kentucky River, resplendent with steeples and trees, old buildings and a picturesque bridge.

Back in Louisville, he combined it with earlier exploring he and John Rice had done out to Eminence, and plotted out a 100-mile ride to Gratz and back. This Chat-N-Nibble ride is the most civilized portion of it.

Scenic Anchorage

Turn right out of **Sawyer Park** and follow Freys Hill Road to Evergreen and pop over the hill to turn left onto Osage Road. Meander through the town of **Anchorage**, a jewel in its own right.

Some of us at the newspaper used to do a ride through here that we called the "Tour of the Great and Near Great," because it went past the homes of *Courier-Journal* editor David Hawpe, then-managing editor Steve Ford, and out to Pewee Valley past the abode of former publisher George Gill. A journalist is irreverent.

Turn right on Lucas Lane and then left on Old LaGrange Road, staying on the less-traveled side of the railroad tracks. Old LaGrange soon joins Westport Road, and crosses the tracks onto Reamer Road. Keep on going.

Safety Note: Reamers becomes Old Floydsburg Road, which twists and winds and takes a sharp downturn at about mile 7.4 that can catch you unawares. Club members have wrecked there. Be careful.

Duncan Chapel and the Countryside

Old Floydsburg emerges at KY 1408 right in front of **Duncan Chapel**, which is old itself, and elegant, and a favorite spot for weddings of people who don't want too many guests. (It's small.)

Continue around to the right and then take a left on 1818, also known as Mt. Zion road, which takes you out into the real country. There are barns and old farm houses along here, and high corn in late summer.

I often find myself in a conversation out here about whether that particular odor you pick up from the fields is something they treat crops with, or the ripening corn itself. It's one of the true smells of summer to me.

Turns onto KY 1315 and then KY 53 take you almost to **Ballardsville**, where you turn right on KY 22 and head for **Smithfield**. The main road takes a loop around to the south a few miles past Ballardsville, but the ride route stays straight on the less-trafficky KY 1861, also known as Smithfield Road, for the little town you come to next.

Smithfield

Smithfield is a sort of anomaly. It's just a crossroads with a store at its hub that has been closed for years. But I seldom have cycled through without hearing the sounds of hammers, as people build houses. A few years ago an **ancient grain mill** there was turned into a collection of gift shops.

Stay straight at the crossroads and you'll be on Giltner Road. Turn left when it reaches KY 22 again, and roll on in to Eminence.

Chat Here, and Nibble

The **Chat-N-Nibble**, revered by club members for its homemade pies, its plate lunches and maybe even its smoked pork tenderloin sandwiches as much as for its name, has made this ride a Louisville favorite.

But that name itself does have its draw. Tom Ferguson, husband of restaurant owner Alice Ferguson, said it rolls regularly off the tongues of disk jockeys in all of the towns around, keeping the venerable eatery on peoples' minds.

He said the name Chat-N-Nibble was an entry in a name-the-restaurant contest held by the café's original owners back in the mid-to-late '40s. "Get a free hamburger if you name the restaurant, that sort of thing," Ferguson said. It stuck.

He said the restaurant dates to about 1945, though the building is about 150 years old. Its owned by the Independent Order of Odd Fellows, whose lodge is upstairs.

Alice Ferguson has owned the restaurant for 11 years, but people still come in looking for Boots and Earl Bartons, its longest-term owners.

Tom Ferguson described the cuisine as "plain old country cooking." He said his mother-in-law, Jenny Sharp, makes the pies at home, and Alice makes a special sauce for the tenderloin. "We smoke the pork," he said.

The restaurant has a regular clientele, including a robust after-church crowd on Sundays, and they don't seem to mind being joined by sweaty groups of cyclists. It's open from 6 a.m. to 5 p.m. Monday through Thursday, and Saturday; and from 6 to 8 Friday, and 11 to 2 Sunday.

Downtown Restoration

Apart from the Chat-N-Nibble, there doesn't seem to be a lot going on in Eminence, but Ferguson said that's deceptive. Though **New Castle**, just up KY 55, is the **Henry County seat**, Eminence is the county's largest town, with about 2,300 residents.

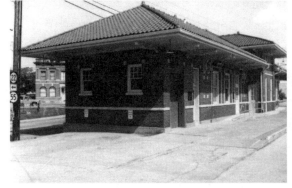

A major downtown restoration project is underway, he said, and many 100-year-old buildings will be restored. An example is the old brick railroad station, on the corner where the route

Eminence's old railroad station, now City Hall

turns down to the restaurant, which has been spruced up and turned into City Hall.

The railroad left Eminence years ago, Ferguson said, but not before it put the town on a path that has kept it Henry County's premiere town for many years.

A Little Backtracking

For purposes of avoiding traffic, the club usually just backtracks through **Smithfield** and up KY 22 to **Ballardsville** for the return trip to Louisville. It's a pretty trip that bears repeating anyway. Just cycle on down Penn Street in front of the restaurant and take the first left, then the first right, then go left on KY 22, and follow Giltner Road and KY 1861.

South of Ballardsville, though, we'll stay on KY 1315 instead of turning back on KY 1818, and ride down to KY 362 and back that way.

The Late, Great, Todds Point Store

There used to be a great little store where 362 meets the road from Simpsonville. Club members would stop there for a soft drink or sometimes a sandwich on various rides in the vicinity, and mingle there with farm folk and others.

There's an old road called Aikens-Anderson Road that takes off toward **Shelbyville** over a hill behind the store, and just a few years ago it used to be exceedingly rural. You saw nothing but barns and fields and old farm houses, though I heard some serious fire and brimstone preaching from a little country church along there as I pedaled by one Sunday morning.

Now the whole road is full of new houses all of the way to Shelbyville. And I don't begrudge the new owners. It must be a great place to live.

But what puzzles me is this: why isn't all of that new population in the area keeping that great little store open?

Trucking on Home

This stretch of 362 is called Todds Point Road, and it's a great, rural, rolling, byway. I love it. A church and a few houses make up the little community of **Todds Point** a mile or so above the store, and then there are farms.

Once my friend Bill Pike and I, on our way back from a hot day's ride to Frankfort, headed out from the store toward some dark clouds in the west. We considered staying at the store until it blew over, but decided we just might beat it home.

It caught us right out on the ridge. Buckets of rain. A deluge. We had to slow way down, but it felt amazingly good. It didn't last long, just cooled us down good and moved on.

Long Run Cut Off

If you chose to start at **Long Run Park**, you will soon recognize KY 1804 on your right—where you turned left earlier and headed down toward Mt. Zion Road. Pass that and you soon come to Long Run Road on your left, and you're nearly back.

There's still some good riding for those of you headed back to Tom Sawyer, though. KY 362 becomes Aiken Road, and dips down through the bed of **Floyds Fork** and crosses a new subdivision around a new golf course.

As this book was going to press, the old one-lane bridge that crossed Floyds Fork was being closed to motor traffic, but bikes were permitted to pass. Officials said it might require circumventing a barrier. The new bridge was expected in two years.

Ride past the old **Avoca depot** and turn right onto Avoca Road.

Safety Note: Be extra careful along Avoca. The route crosses some really rough railroad crossings—presumably kept that way by heavy trucks for a nearby quarry—that can catch a wheel and dump you. Club member Norman Minnick slipped on ice there on a winter ride by himself once and broke a hip.

Ride on through **Anchorage**, turning left on Evergreen, through the Anchorage business district, and head on back out to **Tom Sawyer Park**. If you have thought ahead, you will have some sort of beverage in a cooler in your trunk. You can sit on the grass and talk with your riding companions about what a great trip it was.

(Incidentally, if you've done rides like this a few times, and are looking for that century challenge, here's what you need to know: Ride on out KY 22 from Eminence to Gratz and back—a nice ride—to add 35 miles to the Chat-N-Nibble route.

On the way back from Eminence, stay on KY 53 just after you round the church at Ballardsville, instead of going right onto KY 1315. Hang a right when you get to KY 362 and ride on home through Todds Point. That adds about 5 miles to the route, for a total back at Sawyer of right at 100 miles.)

Route Sheet (1)

0.0	Leave Sawyer Park on Freys Hill Rd.
1.0	Left on Evergreen
2.0	Left on Osage
3.3	Right on Lucas Lane
3.9	Left on Old LaGrange (KY 146)
5.3	Bear right on Westport, straight across tracks and LaGrange onto Reamers Rd.
6.2	Straight on Old Floydsburg
6.3	Cross Ash Road
7.4	Bad downhill - careful
8.0	Straight on KY 1408, past Duncan Chapel and around corner
9.0	Left on KY 1818
14.8	Left on KY 1315
16.3	Left on KY 53
16.9	Right on KY 22, around the church
20.2	Straight on Smithfield Road (KY 1861)
22.1	Smithfield, Ky., straight on Giltner Rd.
25.1	Left on KY 22
27.0	Downtown Eminence, right on KY 55
27.1	Left on S. Penn Ave, to stop at Chat-N-Nibble
27.1	Left on E. Broadway, right on KY 55, Left on KY 22
29.1	Right on Giltner Rd. (KY 1861)
32.2	Smithfield, straight on Smithfield Rd
34.1	Straight on Kentucky 22
37.3	Left on KY 53, at church
37.8	Right on KY 1315
39.4	Straight on KY 1315
43.2	Right on KY 362
44.7	Right on KY 362, by Todds Point Store
49.7	Pass KY 1408
55.7	Right on Avoca
57.9	Right on Evergreen
60.1	Back at park

Route Sheet (2)

<u>Alternate Start from Long Run Park</u>

0.0	Leave park left on Long Run Rd.
1.9	Right on KY 362
2.2	Left on KY 1408
4.1	Right on KY 1818
5.8	Left on KY 1315
7.3	Left on KY 53
7.9	Right on KY 22, around the church
11.2	Straight on Smithfield Rd. (KY 1861)
13.1	Smithfield, Ky., straight on Giltner Rd.
16.1	Left on KY 22
18.0	Downtown Eminence, right on KY 55
18.1	Left on S. Penn Ave, to stop at Chat-N-Nibble
18.1	Left on E. Broadway, right on KY 55, left on KY 22
20.1	Right on Giltner Rd. (KY 1861)
23.2	Smithfield, straight on Smithfield Rd.
25.1	Straight on KY 22
28.3	Left on KY 53, at church
28.8	Right on KY 1315
30.4	Straight on KY 1315
34.2	Right on KY 362
35.7	Right on KY 362, by Todds Point Store
40.7	Pass KY 1408
41.0	Left on Long Run Road
42.8	Long Run Park

Route Sheet (3)

Alternative 2:
Sawyer to Sawyer, by Aiken Road

0.0	Leave Sawyer Park on Freys Hill Rd.
1.0	Left on Evergreen
2.0	Left on Osage
3.3	Right on Lucas Lane
3.9	Left on Old LaGrange (KY 146)
5.3	Bear right on Westport, straight across tracks and LaGrange onto Reamers Rd.
6.2	Straight on Old Floydsburg
6.3	Cross Ash Road
7.4	Bad downhill - careful
8.0	Straight on KY 1408, past Duncan Chapel and around Corner
10.9	Right on KY 362
16.9	Right on Avoca
19.1	Right on Evergreen
21.3	Back at park

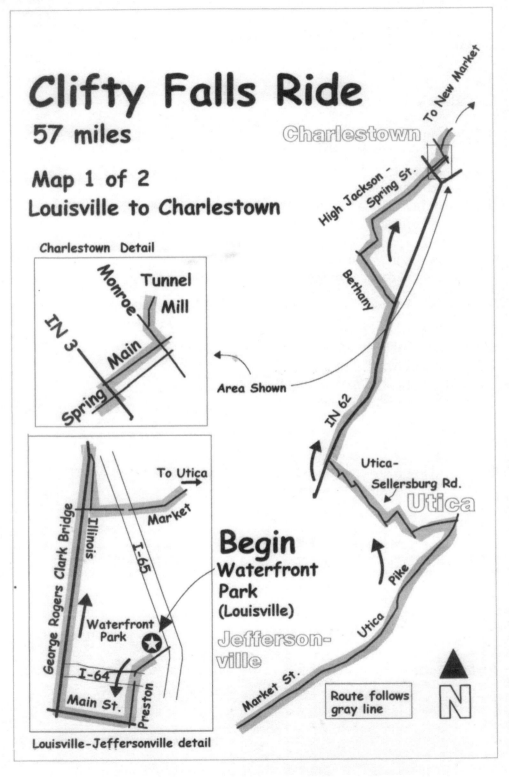

Clifty Falls Ride

57 miles

Map 1 of 2
Louisville to Charlestown

Charlestown

To New Market

High Jackson - Spring St.

Bethany

Charlestown Detail

Monroe

Tunnel Mill

IN 3

Main

Spring

Area Shown

IN 62

Utica-
Sellersburg Rd.

Utica

To Utica

Market

George Rogers Clark Bridge

Illinois

I-65

Begin
Waterfront
Park
(Louisville)

Utica Pike

Waterfront
Park

I-64

Main St.

Preston

Jefferson-
ville

Market St.

Route follows
gray line

N

Louisville-Jeffersonville detail

Clifty Falls Ride

Fifty-seven miles. Numerous hills but no really big ones. Start at Waterfront Park, off River Road near Preston Street.

All of the rides in the book so far have been loops, to make logistics easier. This one is presented as a one-way ride, for which you'll need to arrange return transportation.

But if you do it right, it's a round trip, too, to be done in two days.

It was a favorite ride of Youth Bikers of Louisville, a group of teenagers with whom I and the Louisville bike club had the privilege of being associated for four years in the 1980s. We'd ride up to **Clifty Falls State Park** and other places, camp overnight, and ride back the next day.

The youth group started off as an Explorer Post of the Boy Scouts of America. Some of us in the bike club called the scouts organization, and subsequently reached some interested kids through a newspaper ad.

Among the first to respond was Patti Blair, then 14, who soon became the sparkplug of the group, and remained so for the entire four years. She's Patti Parr now. Philip Rich and his wife, Claudia Foulkes, became the adult leaders, along with me.

Camping

We had an amazingly good time. We'd ride out to a variety of nearby destinations, with Claudia or a parent of one of the young members driving a vehicle to haul tents and baggage and any rider who couldn't make it. We'd stay the night and ride back.

In camp, we would boil up a big pot of spaghetti on a Coleman stove, and toss in some sauce and maybe a little sausage. Those kids would seem to inhale it. Then there was a lot of laughing and joking and some horseplay, but they'd usually turn in fairly early and sleep soundly.

We rode to **General Butler State Park** in Kentucky and to such places as the **West Baden Springs Hotel** in West Baden, Indiana. Sometimes we'd drive to a place and set up camp and then ride out from there, such as **Spring Mill State Park** and **Patoka Lake** in Indiana, and the **Red River Gorge** in Kentucky.

Once the Boy Scouts organization got us a police escort down Dixie Highway through Louisville and Shively for a ride to a camporee at **Fort Knox**. They even blocked intersections.

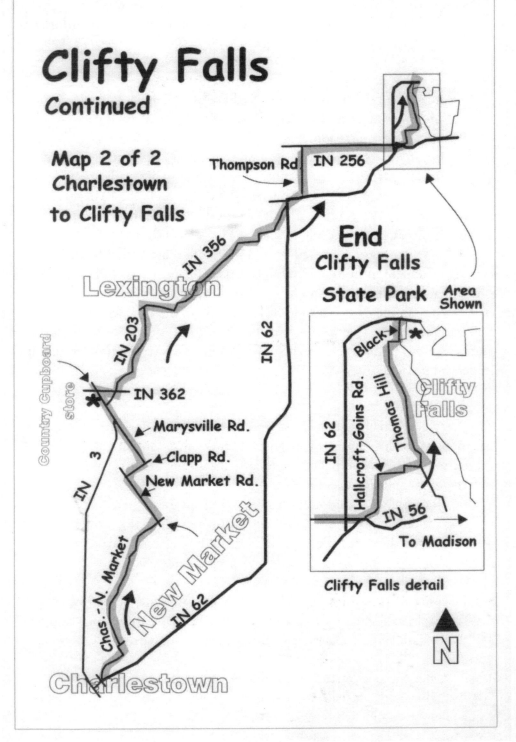

Clifty Falls
Continued

Map 2 of 2
Charlestown
to Clifty Falls

Thompson Rd.   IN 256

IN 356

Lexington

End
Clifty Falls

State Park   Area Shown

IN 203

IN 62

Country Cupboard store

IN 362

Marysville Rd.

Clapp Rd.

New Market Rd.

IN 3

Chas.- N. Market

New Market

IN 62

Black

Clifty Falls

IN 62

Hallcroft–Goins Rd.

Thomas Hill

IN 56

To Madison

Clifty Falls detail

Charlestown

N

My friend Angelo Vaccaro said he happened to get blocked, and he watched in amazement as this small band of cyclists rode through. He said he wondered, "Who the heck are those guys?"

Derby Rides

Anyway, **Clifty Falls** was a favorite of that group, which fluctuated in size from seven or eight to fifteen or so boys and girls through those four summers. We spent several Derby days riding up to Clifty.

The route had been worked out in the '70s by Carol Anderson, a Louisville bike club member who had to drive to the state hospital in Madison occasionally. She was looking for an alternative to IN 62 and US 42 on the Kentucky side.

Each of those is a fairly straight shot up to Madison, and they're still used a lot on club rides. But they can get monotonous, and they were a bit busy for cycling in spots, even then.

Map Matters

I tried mightily to keep all of the rides in this book to one map each. But I couldn't figure out how to portray the detail of both the beginning and the end of this one on a 5.5-inch by 8.5-inch map, and still keep the overall distance in perspective.

Also, I finally decided the trip through Charlestown needed enlarged detail as well. So eventually I just sighed and drew two maps. You follow the Louisville-Jefferson inset on the first map until you get to Market Street in Jeff. Then ride out to Charlestown, and use the Charlestown inset to find your way left on Spring Street—IN 3—right on Main Street past the square, left on Monroe Street, and right on Tunnel Mill Road.

Jump to Map 2 then, and follow it to IN 62 near the park. In the early years, the group pedaled all of the way to the park on that stretch of 62. But it was always a matter of hanging on grimly through none-too-scenic terrain for what seemed like a long time, with cars whizzing by, right at the end of the ride.

The roads in that little chunk of land between 62 and the park complicate the map enough to require an inset, but they keep the rider off the busy road to an arrival point just yards from the park entrance.

Clark Memorial Bridge

We usually started the youth group ride to Clifty from **Crescent Hill**, rode down through Butchertown and along Main Street, and crossed the river on the **Clark Memorial Bridge**—still the only bicycle access Louisville riders have to a lot of very good riding in Southern Indiana.

The bridge may seem like an obstacle to the average inexperienced rider, but club riders use it all of the time. A few years back, city officials made it a little safer by welding iron plates across the expansion joints along the sidewalk on both sides. Otherwise, the joints, especially when expanded, can catch a bicycle wheel and throw a rider down.

Safety Note: That said, I also have to say that I don't think it's very safe to bicycle on the Clark Bridge sidewalks at anything faster than a walking speed, because of conflict with pedestrians, and the danger of hooking a wheel on one of the many heavy girders that intrude on the walkway as you cross.

The speed limit on the bridge is 35 miles an hour. Unfortunately, many motorists seem to regard that as a minimum. Fortunately, the bridge has two lanes in each direction, and motor vehicles will usually move to the center lane to get around cyclists. The right traffic lane is the best place to be, but be careful.

Utica Pike

Double back to your right off the bridge onto Illinois Avenue, and then take a left onto Market Street. From there it's a pretty straight shot out to Utica Pike and Utica, past the **Jeffboat shipyard**, some lovely old riverside houses, and the **Clark Maritime Center** —one of Indiana's largest ports. You get a good glimpse of the mighty Ohio and the Kentucky shore in a few places along there.

In Utica, turn left on Utica-Sellersburg Road, also briefly called Ash Street, right by an old red brick church. Follow Utica-Sellersburg all of the way to IN 62. It makes a few turns along the way, but holds that name through all of them. Follow the route sheet carefully.

You've got almost four miles of IN 62 then, along the old **Army Ammunition Plant** property. It's not the most fun riding, but it's wide and straight. The old plant, where they used to make gunpowder for various wars, is in transition now into an industrial park, called **River Ridge Commerce Center**.

You can see a lot of the old buildings from the road. Most of them will have to be torn down, some because they pose a risk of explosion. There still are powder igloos back in there, though cattle also graze.

Charlestown

After what will seem like quite a long time, you'll spot Bethany Road on the left. It's just after you see a Welcome to Charlestown sign on the right.

Bethany takes you through new subdivisions that were farmland when the youth group used to do this ride, and after a couple of turns, into **Charlestown.**

Go left on Market Street, which is also IN 3, and right at the light on Main Street, past the town square to Monroe Street. Turn left on Monroe and then right on Tunnel Mill Road.

Alternatives

You could make an enjoyable day ride of about 70 miles roundtrip by starting at the town square in Charlestown and following the rest of the map up to Clifty and back.

Woods and Farms

From Tunnel Mill Road, take a left onto Charlestown-New Market Road, and head along some fields and into the woods. It's a great stretch of road. On the left about three miles down that road is an old log house out across a field that intrigues me, though I've never investigated it.

Nearby and closer to the road there's a remarkable replica of a **Swiss chalet.** Soon you come to the little town of New Market at the top of a steep little hill that never fails to catch first-timers in the wrong gear. Pick a low one.

Turn left on New Market Road right at the top of the hill, and cycle past farms and fields to a right turn on Clapp Road, and then a left in Marysville.

Food and Drink

There are a couple of soft drink machines in front of a hardware store on IN 3 in Marysville, but **Kristin's Country Cupboard,** about half a mile up the road, is a good place to get a sandwich and a drink. Hours there are 6 a.m. to 9 p.m. Monday through Saturday, and 6 to 8 Sunday.

A right turn onto IN 362 just after the store takes you on a short hop over to IN 203, where a left turn points you toward Lexington.

Lexington, Indiana

Lexington was a pioneer town that began as a tavern and trading post on the old **Cincinnati Trace,** which was surveyed between Cincinnati and Vincennes, Ind., starting in 1799. That chunk of the trace is now IN 356, which connects Lexington with Madison, and such towns as Vienna, Leota, New Philadelphia and Salem.

There was a newspaper in Lexington by 1815, but the town has depended on Scottsville papers in recent generations. Lexington has a legend about a **lost Indian gold mine,** like the lost silver mine of the Tunnel Mill Road area, based on reported testimony of an Indian named Saskatohawan.

Confederate General **John Hunt Morgan** took Lexington without firing a shot in his 1863 foray through Indiana and Ohio. He spent the night in a local hotel, which is now gone, and left the next day with federal troops in hot pursuit.

Turn right on Main Street in Lexington, IN 356, and ride past the school, which is also the town square, and follow 356 out of town and on about six miles to IN 62.

Riding with Teenagers

The stretch up to IN 62 is a splendid rural one, with a few roller-like hills and nice views of cornfields. Once when I was riding along here with a different group of teenagers—not the club group, but a group from Crescent Hill Baptist Church—a couple of them began complaining that it was too far to Clifty, and too hot, etc.

I told them to quit whining and keep pedaling, and so forth. Then when we got to camp, I found out it actually was 100 degrees out. But they all made it. We all went and jumped in the park pool, which is a short hike from the campground through some cool woods.

Take a left on IN 62 and then a right a couple of tenths of a mile later where IN 56 comes in. The road is headed for **Hanover**, but our route takes a left on Thompson Road, to avoid the Hanover traffic. A couple of rollers later, it takes a right on IN 256.

That stretch is straight as an arrow, and it comes out on IN 62 again, a little over three miles later.

Alternative

If you're not interested in camping, incidentally, you can stay on 256 right across 62, and pedal on down the hill and past the power plant, and into Madison itself. **Madison** is a great town, and only about three miles further—about the same distance as the entrance to the park.

If it's the camping experience you're after, or just a visit to the park before somebody hauls you home, cross IN 62 and then take a left on Hallcroft Drive. Follow it straight onto Goins Road, then take a left on Thomas Hill Road. A right on Black Road will take you out to IN 62, where another right will take you a short distance to the park.

Clifty Falls State Park

It costs $1 for a person on a bike to get into the park, and another $16 for a campsite, or $8 for a primitive campsite. Regular campsites come with access to showers. You can put several tents on a campsite.

If you have a sag wagon—support vehicle—it can get in with drivers and passengers for $4 if it has an Indiana license plate, or $5 if it doesn't.

If you're camping, you still have about 2.3 miles of winding, shady forest road to the campsite. If you're not cooking for yourself, its another couple of miles—the short way—over to the **Clifty Inn**, which has a full service dining room.

Route Sheet

0.0	Right on River Rd. out of Riverfront Park, straight on Preston St.	28.3	Left on New Market Road
		30.5	Right on Clapp Road
		31.3	Left on Marysville Road
0.4	Right on Main St.	33.2	Right on IN 3
0.8	Right on Second St., across the bridge	34.4	Kristin's Country Cupboard
		34.5	Right on IN 362
1.8	Right off bridge, onto Illinois St.	35.2	Left on IN 203
		38.8	Right on Main Street, Lexington (IN 356)
2.0	Left on Market St.	46.0	Left on Indiana 62
5.2	Nice view of the Ohio River	46.2	Right on Indiana 56-62
9.0	Left on Utica-Sellersburg Rd.	46.9	Left on Thompson Road
10.0	Right on Utica-Sellersburg Rd.	48.7	Right on IN 256
		52.2	Cross Ind. 62
10.9	Right on Utica-Sellersburg Rd.	52.4	Left on Hallcroft Drive
		52.7	Stay straight on Goins Road
12.0	Left on Utica-Sellersburg (Don't go into subdivision)	53.6	Left on Thomas Hill Road
12.4	Left on Utica-Sellersburg Rd.	55.7	Right on Black Road
		56.5	Right on IN 62 (park entrance on right)
12.5	Right on Utica-Sellersburg Rd.		
12.8	Right on IN 62, Ammo plant on right		
16.5	Left on Bethany		
17.8	Right on High Jackson Road		
19.8	Past Charlestown Middle School, bear right onto Spring Street		
20.4	Left on Market Street (IN 3)		
20.5	Right on Main Street		
20.9	Left on Monroe Street		
21.0	Right on Tunnell Mill Road		
22.9	Left on Charlestown-New Market Road		
26.0	Old house across the field, Chalet		

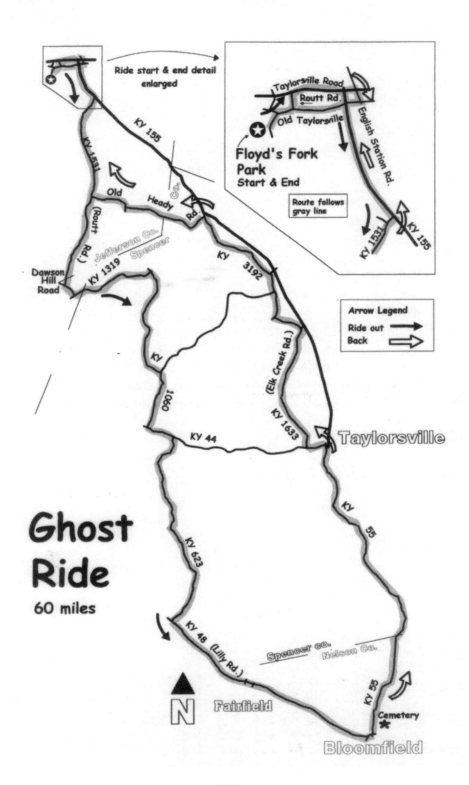

Ride start & end detail enlarged

KY 155

KY 1531

Old
(Routt Rd.)

Heady Rd.

Jefferson Co.
Spencer

KY 1319

Dawson Hill Road

KY 1060

KY 44

KY 3192

(Elk Creek Rd.)

KY 1633

Taylorsville

Floyd's Fork Park
Start & End

Taylorsville Road

Routt Rd.

Old Taylorsville

English Station Rd.

KY 1531

KY 155

Route follows gray line

Arrow Legend
Ride out
Back

KY 55

KY 623

KY 48 (Lilly Rd.)

Spencer Co.
Nelson Co.

KY 55

Cemetery

N

Fairfield

Bloomfield

Ghost
Ride
60 miles

Ghost Ride

Sixty miles. Two significant climbs and some rolling hills. Potential for traffic, especially at start and end. Start at Floyds Fork Park, off Taylorsville Road a mile east of the Gene Snyder Freeway. Turn off Taylorsville Road onto Old Taylorsville Road, and turn south on Pope Lick Road into the Park.

Back in the '80s when the club had a group of teenage cyclists that would go on overnight bicycle camping trips, we used to tell ghost stories at night. I had one about a high-wheel cyclist back in the the 1880s who got separated from fellow riders on a Louisville to Bardstown ride. He found himself outside of Taylorsville, headed for Bloomfield, wondering if he might be lost.

So he decided to stop and ask a woman he saw walking up the road ahead of him. When he got closer, and down off his big wheel, he noticed she was strange. Her clothes, though of good quality, were out of date, and she was pale with an odd look in her eye.

When he asked if she could tell him the way to Bardstown, she didn't seem to comprehend. She just said, "I must return to the arms of my good husband."

She repeated it when he asked again. He concluded there was something wrong with her, and decided to ride on and let somebody at the next farm house know she was out there.

Odd Recurrence

A couple of hills later, though, he saw another person walking, and at closer range it looked very much like the same woman. And before he could even speak, she said, "I must return to the arms of my good husband."

It was too spooky for him. He rode on, determined to put distance between himself and her. He saw her again on another rise ahead of him, and was trying to decide what to do, when she moved up a path away from the road. He got to the path, and saw that it led to a graveyard.

It was starting to get dark and he knew he should press on, but he had to find out what was going on. So he stashed his wheel and followed her a way, and she seemed to vanish near some older graves to the right of the path.

He walked to where he'd last seen her, and found a flat stone with a long inscription. It made the hair stand up on the back of his neck.

"Entomb'd within each other's arms," it began,

"The husband and the wife repose
Safe from life's never-ending storms
And safe from all their cruel foes."

There was a good deal more, but the cyclist ran back down the path, grabbed his bike, and rode on to Bloomfield, which was only a short distance.

History Lesson

We'll get to what happened next in a minute, but you need to know that the story was a setup. **Bloomfield** is on the Louisville club's Old Kentucky Home Tour, which we would take the youth group on. And Bloomfield is the keeper of an 1826 story about a tragic love triangle—that of Anna Cook, Jeroboam O. Beauchamp, and Solomon Sharp, who was speaker of the Kentucky House of Representatives.

I figured it would appeal to teenagers.

But first, about the ride.

Old Kentucky Home

This ride takes in some of the roads of the Louisville club's Old Kentucky Home Tour, known affectionately as the The Bardstown Ride, or OKHT. It was coming up on its 25th year as this was being written, and 900 to 1,000 riders were expected. They ride to Bardstown on a September day, stay over night, and ride back the next day.

Actually, I maintain that the ride started in 1977 when *The Courier-Journal* sponsored a bike trip to Bardstown, thinking it would copy the Des Moines newspaper's great success with the Register's Annual Great Bicycle Ride Across Iowa, also known as RAGBRAI. The *C-J* ride drew almost 300 people.

But the *Courier* gave up after that first year, and the bike club sponsored a Bardstown ride the next year. My friend Stewart Prather, who was club president then, claims it was just a coincidence that the club ride went to the same town.

But it doesn't matter. In any case, the OKHT has grown and prospered. Riders have their choice of three routes down to Bardtown, including a relatively easy 55-miler and a grueling 100-mile ride with some huge hills.

There is another 55-mile route back to Louisville, which everybody takes the second day. It is beautiful. To get the real effect of the Bardstown ride, with great food at sag stops and the camaraderie of those hundreds of riders, you really have to do the club ride.

This ride attempts to give you a taste of the route, by combining a bit of the easy ride down and a chunk of the ride back with a stop at the Bloomfield graveyard.

Map Matters

To keep mileage down on this round trip ride, I start at **Floyd Fork Park** off Taylorsville Road about a mile east of the **Gene Snyder Freeway**.

The beginning of the ride is easy to do, but a bit hard to describe, as a glance at the map will suggest. It follows part of the old Tour de Gil ride, which used to come down Routt Road by the park, over a now-defunct bridge across the **Floyds Fork** of the Salt River.

But the bridge was gone as this was written, and that complicated my map. To get to the main part of Routt Road, you had to use a chunk of KY 155 to get across the fork. And to do that, you had to use a short stretch of Taylorsville Road, which can be busy.

As a practical matter, that's fairly easy to do on the outbound trip, because it's a short distance to 155, and you don't have to cross any traffic.

Retracing that exact route on the return trip, though, would involve a couple of turns across traffic. The club often chooses to avoid that by using a roundabout—but still short—return route.

You come down the hill on KY 155 and take a right instead of a left, and then take the short trip to English Station Road, and double back to the park on Old Taylorsville Road.

It's easy enough to ride, as I said, but a bit complicated to map, especially if you're trying to keep the map small enough for a stem clip. I tried to help by pulling the start detail out into an enlarged inset. But it still might help to look at the map and the route sheet a bit before starting out. At press time there were plans to rebuild the Routt Road bridge, perhaps in a year.

Routt Road, the Country Pantry and Plum Creek

Anyway, take 155 to the top of the hill, take a right, and get onto Routt Road. Follow it all the way to Dawson Hill Road and take a left. **The Country Pantry** is just a few hundred yards left, and it's a good place to get a soft drink or a snack.

It's open from 5 a.m. to 9 p.m. Monday through Friday, from 7 to 9 on Saturday, and from 8 to 7 on Sunday.

Turn left on KY 1319 and follow it down the long winding hill to KY 1060. Turn right to follow another winding road along **Plum Creek**—always a favorite stretch of Bardstown riders. A left turn on KY 44 takes you over the hill to another right turn on KY 623.

And that takes you across the **Salt River**, and up what is eventually going to strike you as a fairly significant hill. It comes on you kind of gradually, and you might not notice it at first. Shift way down.

A left on Lilly Road—also KY 48—takes you into Fairfield, where you can stop at **Joy's Grocery**. It's open from 5 a.m. to 9 p.m. Monday through Friday, from 6:30 to 9 Saturday, and from 7:30 to 7 on Sunday.

The Love Story

Another four miles and you're in **Bloomfield**. Take a left on Hill Street and another on KY 55, and climb a short distance to the **cemetery**.

About that love story. In Bloomfield, the 1880s rider was told that he'd seen the grave of Jeroboam Beauchamp and his wife, Anna, and he learned their sad story. Beauchamp was a young lawyer from the Bowling Green area, who fell in love with Anna even though she was 16 years older than he. And Anna had history. She'd been involved some years earlier with Solomon Sharp, another attorney and a rising politician. Sharp abandoned her, and there was a child, and it died.

She wanted her honor avenged. Beauchamp agreed to do that, and they were married. He took a trip to Frankfort and knocked on Sharp's door one dark night, and stabbed him in the heart. He was immediately suspected of the crime, and soon convicted. Anna talked her way into his cell the night before he was to hang, and they planned a joint suicide.

She succeeded, but he was patched up enough to go to the gallows on schedule. It was July 7, 1826. Anna had previously arranged with Beauchamp relatives at Bloomfield that they'd be buried in the same grave, and that a long poem she wrote would be chiseled on a flat stone that covered their resting place.

Historic Site

The grave is still there, though the original stone is broken and hard to read. A few years ago, a new upright stone was added, with the poem newly-chiseled. And there's a state historic marker telling all about it out on the road.

The youth group riders always wanted to stop.

Taylorsville and Elk Creek

The route takes you on to **Taylorsville**, down a nice long hill where you cross the Salt River again. Take a left on KY 44, and a right on 1633, which is Elk Creek Road. You'll come to a bit of a hill, climbing up a nice, shady gorge, in a few miles. It's real good practice.

Turn left to stay on 1633, and left again on KY 3192 at Elk Creek, and take another left onto Old Heady Road. For some reason, Old Heady always makes me feel like I'm riding in New England. It sounds vaguely colonial, some way.

Old Heady takes you back to Routt Road, where you turn right and retrace your pedaling back to KY 155 at the top of the hill, and coast practically all of the way back to the start.

Remember to turn right at Taylorsville Road, and right again on English Station and then on Old Taylorsville Road, to double back under the highway and head back for the park. A left on Pope Lick Road gets you there.

Route Sheet

0.0	Leave parking lot at Floyds Fork Park	29.7	Left on KY 55
		30.0	Graveyard
0.1	Left on Pope Lick Road	39.3	Left on KY 44 in Taylorsville
0.3	Right on Old Taylorsville Road	39.8	Right on KY 1633, Elk Creek Road
0.4	Left on Routt Road	41.1	Big, twisty hill
0.5	Right on Taylorsville Road	43.6	Left to stay on KY 1633
1.0	Right on KY 155	45.7	Left on KY 3192
2.2	Right on KY 1531	48.5	Left on Old Heady Road
8.0	Left on Dawson Hill Road	52.2	Right on Routt Road
8.5	Left on KY 1319	55.3	Left on KY 155
10.9	Right on KY 1060	56.5	Right on Taylorsville Road
16.0	Left on KY 44	56.8	Right on English Station Road
16.8	Right on KY 623		
22.8	Left on Lilly Road	56.9	Right on Old Taylorsville Road
25.7	Joy's Grocery		
29.6	Left on Hill Street in Bloomfield	57.9	Left on Pope Lick
		58.1	Right into park

Bloomington Trail Ride
90/67 miles

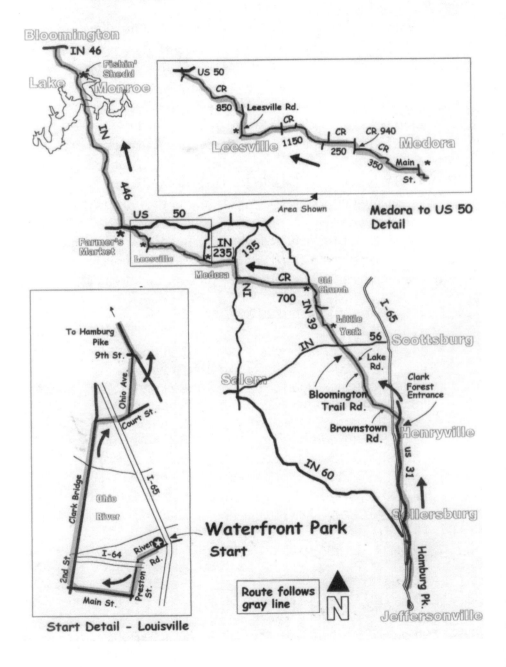

Bloomington
IN 46
Fishin' Shedd
Lake Monroe
IN
446

Medora to US 50 Detail

US 50
CR 850
Leesville Rd.
CR
Leesville
CR 1150
CR 250
CR 940
CR 350
Medora
Main St.

Area Shown

Farmer's Market
US 50
Leesville
IN 235
IN 135
Medora
IN
CR 700
Old Church
IN 39
Little York
I-65
56
Scottsburg
IN
Salem
Lake Rd.
Bloomington Trail Rd.
Clark Forest Entrance
Brownstown Rd.
Henryville
IN 60
us 31
Sellersburg
Hamburg Pk.
Jeffersonville

Start Detail - Louisville

To Hamburg Pike
9th St.
Ohio Ave.
Court St.
Clark Bridge
Ohio River
I-65
I-64
2nd St.
River Rd.
Preston St.
Main St.
Waterfront Park Start

Route follows gray line

N

Bloomington Trail

Ninety miles, or 67 miles. Some hills, but only one significant one. Some traffic possible in the early going. Potential for high water problems in springtime. Start at Waterfront Park, which is off River Road near its intersection with Preston Street.

When my daughter, Senlin, did the Old Kentucky Home ride to Bardstown with me at age 10, she marveled that we had left Louisville without a car, and still had arrived in "a whole different town." If you've been doing as I suggested, and working up to longer rides, your bike will have given you a good bit of motor-free mobility too, by the time you get to this point.

And this ride, the last in the book, is intended to celebrate that mobility by taking you to a whole 'nother town.

Bloomington, home of Indiana University, my alma mater, is a marvelous place, but we won't dwell on it. For this ride, the trip's the thing.

Century Time

Though I give you 90 and 67-mile options when measured roughly from the Ohio River in Louisville to the junction of IN 446 and IN 46 in Bloomington, this is really a 100-mile ride, if you do it right.

My friend Bill Pike says that doing a ride "right" means no auto involvement—that a ride is somehow tainted if it doesn't start at your door. I used to leave my door in Crescent Hill for this ride, and my odometer would just turn over 100 when I arrived at my mother-in-law's door in Bloomington. So, depending on where you start and what your destination is in Bloomington, you could arrange that, too.

I've set the formal start of the ride at **Waterfront Park**, because it has parking, and is near the **Clark Memorial Bridge**, the traditional early morning meeting place of Louisville club members intent on riding to Bloomington in the fall to do the Hilly Hundred invitational ride.

Some of you readers probably could start at your own houses, if you wanted to.

I've put the formal end at **Bruster's Old Fashioned Ice Cream & Yogurt Shop** on IN 46 in Bloomington, which I recommend. You could arrange for some other destination.

175

Alternatives

It's good to start this ride early in the morning, for a couple of reasons. One is that it's a long way, and you might want to dawdle as you go. Another is that some of the roads in the early going can get crowded when business and commuter traffic pick up, and that can make riding less fun.

While Bill Pike is right and there is something to be said for door-to-door biking, there also is something to be said for just getting out and riding your bike without worrying too much about hurtling hunks of "Detroit Iron," as the Critical Mass riders like to say.

So, if you don't mind sacrificing that complete city-to-city feeling, this ride is entirely startable at **Clark County State Forest**, on US 31, just north of Henryville, Ind. You can leave a car in the parking lot, a few hundred yards from where the really country part of this ride starts.

That would get you past the traffic of Jeffersontown and Hamburg Pike, and through Sellersburg and Henryville on US 31. You will miss some good stuff, but not that much.

If you don't plan to ride back—and that has been done—someone will have to drive up to get you. That person could just drop you off at the Forest and go on to Bloomington while you ride your bicycle.

Map Matters

It is, as I said, a long way to Bloomington, and some of the details of getting out of Riverfront Park for starters, and later for navigating the many county roads between Medora and US 50, made a couple of insets necessary on the map for this ride.

It should be easy enough to follow, though. Just start with the Louisville inset and pick up the main map on Spring St. and Hamburg Pike in Jeffersonville. When you head out of Medora for that nice after-lunch climb, check out the Medora inset.

Second Street Bridge

If you start out in Riverfront Park and take Preston Street to Main Street, then Main to Second Street, you come to the Clark Memorial Bridge, which I mentioned earlier on the Clifty Falls Ride.

It may seem a bit daunting to the inexperienced rider, but club riders use it all of the time. Just consider it another street. Stay to the right, where there are iron plates welded in place to keep your tires out of expansion joints, and pedal on across.

Jeffersonville

Once you clear the bridge, the next chore is to thread your way under I-65 on Court Street. After you've passed through the traffic light just east of the highway, work your way to the left lane and watch for Ohio Avenue a few yards east on Court. Ohio usually is not too busy, especially early.

Ohio leads you into an intersection at 9th Street, where you jog right, and then turn left on Spring Street. Watch for oncoming traffic on 9th as you make that maneuver. Then just stay on Spring until it becomes Hamburg Pike, and eventually turns onto US 31.

Sellersburg

At Sellersburg, US 31 makes a turn to the left, and then a right turn at a stop light. That's not a bad route to take early in the day.

If you find yourself under traffic pressure there, though, it's easy to thread your way through town on alternate streets. Just stay straight on Penn St. where U.S. 31 turns left. There was no Penn Street sign at the intersection when I was writing this book, but the way is obvious.

Take that down to East Utica Street and turn left. Then turn right on Indiana Street, which is the local designation for that stretch of US 31.

Clark County State Forest

It's about 10 miles on to Henryville, then, and another mile or so to the entrance to **Clark County State Forest.** If you've been riding from Louisville, notice how good it feels to be all warmed up with 20 miles under your belt, and ready after some urban cycling for a nice sojourn in the woods.

You turn left at Brownstown Road. Somewhere, as it twists and climbs and coasts through farmsteads and residential areas just outside the forest, it becomes Bloomington Trail Road.

It used to be Bloomington Trail, a main wagon and saddle horse route from Louisville, through Bloomington, to Indianapolis. An 1884 history of several southern Indiana counties mentions that in the early 1800s there was a famous **Inn at Little York**, where wagon drivers could get food and drink and entertainment.

Think what those drivers and other travelers would have thought if they'd known you would come pedaling through town some day, fully under your own power, on a metal machine not much heavier than a good saddle, having come all the way from Louisville and confident of making Bloomington with plenty of daylight left.

Leota

First, though, you get through **Leota**, a small place many a cyclist has visited mostly for the sound of the name. "Leotee," some in the vicinity say. Note old cemeteries and other attractions along the way.

You take the right fork immediately out of the covered bridge at Leota. There is one tricky spot on Bloomington Trail a couple of miles north of there, where it inexplicably changes its name to W. Lake Road, and turns left at a stop sign.

It remains Lake Road for only one tenth of a mile, then curves to the right and becomes Bloomington Trail again. If you miss that turn and find yourself on Zion Road, you can continue north across IN 56, and turn left on Little York Road and get to Little York just the same, by an equally lovely route. But it's longer.

Little York

Bloomington Trail reaches IN 56 just where IN 39 comes south from Little York. You cross and go straight into that historic but very small community. The 1884 history book says early settlers from New York gave the town its name, but it doesn't say much else.

A few years ago, a new **livestock sales facility** was built near Little York and it is considered a successor to Louisville's venerable **Bourbon Stockyards**, which closed in 1999 after 165 years in operation. Some Little York citizens opposed it, but area farmers tired of hauling cows to Indianapolis put up $100,000 toward building it.

Old Dutch Church

The ride from Louisville to Bloomington evolved over the years. Some of the first rides went from Hamburg up IN 60 to Salem, then north

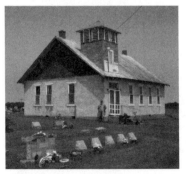

on IN 135. Later, we started staying on US 31, sometimes as far as Scottsburg, and taking various routes west. Sometimes we wandered a bit.

There's an **old church** at the corner of IN 39 and County Road 700 that became a landmark for a left turn over to IN 135. It is vaguely European in appearance—sort of Dutch, somebody on one of those early rides

The "old Dutch Church"

thought —and a turn at "the Old Dutch Church" became a part of lore for the Bloomington ride.

Actually, it's called **Russell Chapel Church**. I was going by one day, and spotted Charles Combs, the church's 77-year-old caretaker, on his lawn tractor. He said the church was built in 1923 on the site of two earlier houses of worship, one of which "blew into the field over there," and the other a victim of fire.

As this book was written the church had "eight, ten, or twelve" members, and was non-denominational, having given up an affiliation with Methodists when they wanted to shut it down.

Combs said it was built of tile blocks covered with stucco, unlikely to burn *or* blow into the field. It has a tin roof. The stucco had cracked away in spots, showing the brick-red tile underneath.

Round Barn

County Road 700 goes almost straight west to IN 135. You can tell when you are almost there by an old round barn, which is on 135 just past the corner. The husband of the woman who owns the barn with her brothers told me it was built about 1902 and still was used for livestock, though it was getting expensive to maintain.

As I was talking to him, a sport utility vehicle carrying two women slowed for a look at the barn, and the driver said, "Isn't that a marvelous surprise?"

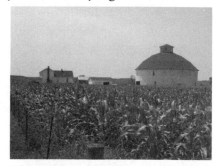

It's actually quite famous. It's called the **Burcham Round Barn**, one of three in Jackson County, and of about 100 in Indiana. It's listed as a county tourist attraction.

The Burcham Round Barn

Covered Bridge

The turn off IN 135 is just a couple of miles up the road. IN 235 takes you over to the small town of **Medora**, which notes in *its* list of tourist attractions that **John Cougar Mellencamp**, from nearby **Seymour, Ind.**, filmed a video called "Hurts so Good" there in 1984.

A slogan for a long bike ride if I ever heard one.

Before you get to town, though, notice the **covered bridge** just off IN 235 where it crosses the East Fork of the **White River**. That's the **longest covered bridge in the U.S.**, according to Jackson County officials.

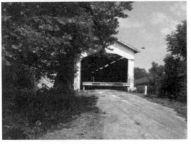

Covered bridge built in 1875

It's 458 feet long when you consider the 12-foot overhangs, the county says. It was built in 1875, and it carried traffic on IN 235 into Medora until 1972, just five years before I first rode into town.

The flat, low land between the bridge and town floods in wet weather —as do some stretches of the aforementioned County Road 700, something to keep in mind if you're planning a trip in the spring of the year.

Roads in this part of Indiana have flooded for years. I found an account in an 1896 *Courier-Journal* of a man exploring by bike who was "obliged to undress and carry his wheel on his head for a considerable distance."

There's a big ride through Iowa where people do that sort of thing, but it's because they're drunk.

Catfish and Beer

Medora is best known to cyclists on the ride to Bloomington as a good place to stop for lunch. For some years, a group of us would get catfish sandwiches there, and share a pitcher of beer.

The place where we did it is still there, though under new management, and called **The Legendary Perry Street Tavern.** You could still get fish sandwiches there, along with steaks and plate lunches.

Owner Tim Davers said the place is open from "9 a.m. to closing," which I gathered is likely to be in the wee hours. You also can get food and drink at the **Medora Dairy Bar**, open 10 a.m. to 9:30 p.m. every day but Sunday, when it's closed.

Randy's Market, a grocery on Main Street where you turn left to head for County Road 350, serves sandwiches and soft drinks and sells such snacks as peanut butter and cheese crackers. It's open 8-7 most days, 9-5 on Sunday. Randy's, which is in an old building with wide, unfinished but freshly swept pine floorboards, also has a great collection of old photographs on one wall.

Medora Hill

The first thing you will notice going west out of Medora, after Main Street becomes County Road 350, is a fairly significant hill. You'll need to go to a low gear here, and grind away.

Hills are good for you, as I have said. And this one is well worth it, because this route, which I discovered with a Louisville Bicycle Club youth group once when we were riding out of nearby **Spring Mill State Park**, is a vast improvement over the way we used to go, which was up IN 235 and across a long stretch of US 50.

It's a moderately tough practice hill, but very doable. People have done it while digesting catfish and beer, though I don't actually do that myself anymore.

From the top of the hill, you're into a sort of labyrinth of county roads. Follow the map or route sheet carefully. The roads are small, with a lot of turns and branches, through hill-type farm country, really off the beaten path.

I was annoyed to discover recently that a bunch of county dumpsters that used to tell me where to turn onto County Road 850 north of Leesville have been removed. The county thoughtfully replaced them with a "No Dumping Allowed" sign, though. So turn there.

Follow CR 850 up to US 50, and turn left for a short ride to IN 446.

Long Lonesome Road

There's a store called **Farmer's Market** on US 50, right at its intersection with IN 446, that deserves consideration for a stop. You won't see another store for 17 miles.

The market, a sort of service-station-convenience-store-restaurant, is owned by a family named Farmer, and is not to be confused with a place where you buy vegetables. Fried food seems more the main fare. But you can buy soft drinks and snacks, and get a sandwich from the meat case.

It's open from 5 a.m. to 9 p.m. Monday through Friday, and 6 to 9 Sunday.

IN 446 takes you across **Lake Monroe** to **Bloomington**, and it is a great road—wide and smooth, without too many hills. But it goes through sections of the **Hoosier National Forest**, and aside from farms, there is not much civilization along it.

By this time you also are getting quite a few miles in, and rest and drinks are seeming like a better and better idea. There used to be a bait shop a couple of miles south of the lake. I never did this ride with a group that didn't want to stop there.

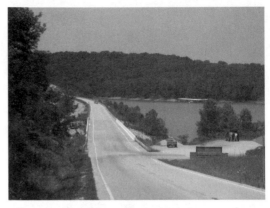

Causeway across Monroe Reservoir

But that shop, whose owner once told us it was a favorite hangout of then-IU basketball coach **Bobby Knight**, has closed.

So you have to go on to the **Fishin' Shedd**, almost three miles up the road toward Bloomington after you cross the lake. It sells soft drinks, snacks and pre-made sandwiches. It opens at 5 a.m. every day, and closes at 8:30 p.m. Monday through Thursday, 9 p.m. Friday and Saturday, and 8 p.m. Sunday.

From there, it's just a short shot up to Bloomington, where it's good to stop pedaling. If you have previously arranged for a place to take a shower and drink a beer—as I used to do when I got to my mother-in-law's place in Bloomington—it is good.

Route Sheet

0.0	Leave Waterfront Park		65.4	Left on US 50
0.4	Right on Main Street		66.3	Right on IN 446. Farmer's Market store
0.8	Right on Second Street, across the bridge		81.9	Cross causeway at Lake Monroe
2.1	Right off bridge onto Court St		83.4	Fishin' Shedd store
2.3	Left on Ohio Avenue		89.5	Arrive at IN 46 in Bloomington
2.7	Jog right on 9th Street and turn left on Spring Street			

0.0 Leave Waterfront Park
0.4 Right on Main Street
0.8 Right on Second Street, across the bridge
2.1 Right off bridge onto Court St
2.3 Left on Ohio Avenue
2.7 Jog right on 9th Street and turn left on Spring Street
3.5 Straight on Hamburg Pike
8.0 Right on US 31
10.1 Bear left on US 31
11.0 Right on US 31 in Sellersburg (Alternative to the above two turns: Straight on Penn Street, left on Utica Street, right on Indiana, which is US 31)
22.7 Left on Brownstown Road, which becomes Bloomington Trail Road
30.3 Right on Bloomington Trail out of bridge at Leota
32.1 Left on W. Lake Road (becomes Bloomington Tr.)
33.4 Right on IN 39, cross IN 56
36.3 Right on Scifero Road (local name for a section of IN39)
38.8 Cross IN 256
41.3 Left on CR 700 (at "Dutch" church)
49.8 Right on IN 135
51.8 Left on IN 235
53.6 Right on IN 235 in Medora
53.8 Left on Main Street (Becomes CR 350)
55.0 Big hill
56.3 Right on CW 940
56.5 Left on CW 250
58.8 Left on CR 1150
62.8 Right onto Leesville Road at Leesville
63.5 Left on CR 850 by no dumping sign
65.4 Left on US 50
66.3 Right on IN 446. Farmer's Market store
81.9 Cross causeway at Lake Monroe
83.4 Fishin' Shedd store
89.5 Arrive at IN 46 in Bloomington

Alternate

0.0 Leave Clark County Forest
0.3 Left on Brownstown Road, which becomes Bloomington Trail Road
7.9 Right on Bloomington Trail out of bridge at Leota
9.7 Left on W. Lake Road (Becomes Bloomington Trail)
11.0 Right on IN 39, cross IN 56
12.6 Right on Scifero Road (local name for a section of IN39)
15.1 Cross IN 256
17.6 Left on CR 700 (at "Dutch" church)
26.1 Right on IN 135
28.1 Left on IN 235
29.9 Right on IN 235 in Medora
30.1 Left on Main Street (becomes CR 350)
31.3 Big hill
32.6 Right on CW 940
32.8 Left on CW 250
35.1 Left on CR 1150
39.1 Right onto Leesville Road in Leesville
40.8 Left on CR 850 by no dumping sign
42.7 Left on US 50
43.6 Right on IN 446. Farmers Market store
59.2 Cross causeway at Lake Monroe
61.7 Fishin' Shedd store
66.8 Arrive at IN 46 in Bloomington

My Trip Journal

Date:
Tour, Route or Location:

_____

_____

_____

_____

_____

_____

_____

_____

_____

_____

_____

_____

_____

_____

_____

_____

_____

_____

_____

_____

_____

_____

_____

_____

My Trip Journal

Date:
Tour, Route or Location:

My Trip Journal

Date:
Tour, Route or Location:

My Trip Journal

Date:
Tour, Route or Location:

My Trip Journal

Date:
Tour, Route or Location:

My Trip Journal

Date:
Tour, Route or Location:

My Trip Journal

Date:
Tour, Route or Location:

_____

_____

_____

_____

_____

_____

_____

_____

_____

_____

_____

_____

_____

_____

_____

_____

_____

_____

_____

_____

_____

_____

_____

_____

_____

_____

_____

My Trip Journal

Date:
Tour, Route or Location:

My Trip Journal

Date:
Tour, Route or Location: